WHAT PEOPLE ARE SAYING ABOUT

YOU CAN BEAT LUNG CANCER

This is one of the most comprehensive books available on alternative treatments for lung cancer. It explains the treatments used successfully by a health professional/cancer survivor of 38 years and by some of the leading medical and health practitioners currently in the field. It will be useful, not just for the lay reader, but also for therapists and others with a scientific background.

G. Edward Griffin, Author of *World Without Cancer, The Politics of Cancer Therapy,* and other books and films. Recipient of the Telly Award for Excellence in Television Production. President of American Media.

Carl Helvie's case is remarkable. This is a man of great courage, who has followed a natural approach to his life-threatening illness and this has resulted in a cure. This has to be impressive and his book deserves a wide readership, which I hope it will get.

Julian Kenyon, MD, Medical Director, The Dove Clinic for Integrated Medicine, London & Winchester, Founder President of the British Society of Integrated Medicine

Lung cancer is both common and lethal. Dr. Helvie approaches this subject as both a health care professional and a lung cancer survivor. This book is extremely readable for all cancer patients and holds invaluable advice for beating this disease that is often called "a death sentence" if diagnosed in later stages of the disease. Dr. Helvie has not only offered his invaluable experiences as a cancer victor, but adds the wisdom of other world-class experts on the subject of cancer treatment. If you or a loved one has lung cancer, then this book could become your 'get out of jail free' card toward recovery or at least a dramatic extension in quality and quantity of life.

Patrick Quillin, PhD, RD, CNS; Author of *Beating Cancer with Nutrition* and *Adjuvant Nutrition in Cancer Treatment*, Organizer of 3 scientific symposia on nutrition and cancer

If you are ever diagnosed with advanced cancer, the odds are very good that your oncologist will tell you that unless you immediately consent to chemotherapy you are going to die. This is a lie! I know, I have been treating conventional chemotherapy failures for years. Other than for leukemia or lymphoma, conventional chemotherapy is almost always a death sentence. There are so many more effective ways to treat advanced cancer, and Dr. Carl Helvie's book, *You Can Beat Lung Cancer: Using Alternative/Integrative Interventions*, describes some of the most effective. In addition, his book is packed with references and information sources that will help anyone fighting cancer learn more about how to go about it successfully

Frank Shallenberger, MD, HMD, ABAAM

Medical Director, The Nevada Center of Alternative Medicine, Editor, Real Cures Newsletter, Author, *The Type-2 Diabetes Breakthrough, Principles and Applications of Ozone Therapy,* and *Bursting With Energy*

This is an excellent book! It is both a resource and an inspiration for cancer patients and their loved ones and caregivers.

Richard Linchitz, MD, Medical Director, Linchitz Medical Wellness, Author of *Life Without Pain*

This is a valuable piece of writing, to give people hope that there are other ways back to health from cancer, than the 'slash, burn and poison' offered by conventional oncology.

Robert A. Eslinger, DO, HMD, Medical Director, Reno Integrative Medical Center

In this fine book, *You Can Beat Lung Cancer: Using Alternative/ Integrative Interventions,* Carl Helvie shares how he cured himself of his incurable cancer. Interested yet? The reader will appreciate practical advice on the biochemical, the nutritional and the spiritual factors which create health. I have been priviledged to care for people with terminal cancer for over 20 years and agree with Carl that the best approach is to nourish the person, not attack the cancer. Common sense strategies so lacking in health care today can be found in these pages: culivate a habit of service, create purpose in life, detoxify, replenish and support vitality.

Bradford S. Weeks, M.D. The Weeks Clinic for Corrective Health, www.weeksclinic.com www.weeksmd.com www.correc tivehealth.org

Carl Helvie's insightful journey through the terror of a diagnosis of lung cancer, usually a death sentence, shows us how we have an internal guidance system that can steer us through "the valley of the shadow of death". His story is also that of the archetype of the wounded healer who emerges from a serious life-threatening illness with insights to help others facing similar challenges. With these new insights, healers such as Carl change the paradigm for the human race by rewriting the outcome of what before were nearly always fatal diseases. These wounded healers show us what is possible when we wake up to who we truly are.

Susan E. Kolb MD, FACS, ABIHM. Author of *The Naked Truth About Breast Implants.* Contributing author *Goddess Shift: Women Leading for a Change* and *Optimism!* by Stephanie Marohn.

We at the Life Extension Foundation field thousands of calls a year from cancer patients seeking alternatives to toxic FDA approved therapies. We are always pleasantly surprised when a cancer victim turns into a cancer victor by going outside the mainstream to aggressively implement multi-modal approaches to eradicate their disease. There is tremendous individual variability with each cancer case, meaning that alternative therapies can play an important role not only in mitigating toxic conventional treatment side effects, but also suppressing survival factors that enable cancer cells to escape destruction.

William Faloon, Co-Founder, Life Extension Foundation

You Can Beat Lung Cancer

Using Alternative/Integrative
Interventions

You Can Beat Lung Cancer

Using Alternative/Integrative
Interventions

Carl O. Helvie, RN, DrPH

(A 38 Year Survivor)

With Additions By: Bernie Siegel, MD;
Francisco Contreras, MD;
James Forsythe MD, HMD;
Kim Dalzell, PhD, RD;
and Tanya Harter Pierce, MA, MFCC

AYNI
BOOKS

Winchester, UK
Washington, USA

First published by Ayni Books, 2012
Ayni Books is an imprint of John Hunt Publishing Ltd., Laurel House, Station Approach,
Alresford, Hants, SO24 9JH, UK
office1@jhpbooks.net
www.johnhuntpublishing.com

For distributor details and how to order please visit the 'Ordering' section on our website.

Text copyright: Carl O. Helvie 2011

ISBN: 978 1 78099 283 9

A CIP catalogue record for this book is available from the British Library.

Design: Stuart Davies

Printed in the USA by Edwards Brothers Malloy

We operate a distinctive and ethical publishing philosophy in all
areas of our business, from our global network of authors to
production and worldwide distribution.

CONTENTS

This book is dedicated to those individuals who have
Successfully used alternative, natural, noninvasive
Cancer interventions in the past:
Those brave physicians who have provided them,
And others choosing to use them in the future.

A Message from the Author

Please keep in mind that cancer, health, environment, and relationship information is an ever-changing process. As new research broadens our knowledge in these areas, changes in prevention and treatment follow. The author of this work has checked with sources believed to be reliable in his effort to provide information that is complete, accurate, and reliable.

However, in view of the possibility of human error or changes in research findings, neither the author nor the publisher nor any other party who has been involved in the preparation or publication of the work is responsible for any errors or omissions or for the results obtained from the use of such information. Readers are encouraged to confirm the information contained herein with other sources.

Introduction

My First Experience with Cancer

Over 60 years ago my mother was diagnosed with the big C as cancer was known at that time. It was a frightening diagnosed and a disease that affected many people. My mother left home to spent time in a hospital that was over one hundred miles away. There she received invasive treatment that destroyed both the cancer cells and the surrounding normal cells. Fortunately, she survived the ordeal and lived many more years. I believe her survival was mainly a result of her faith and optimism. When she returned home, our family doctor told her he had not believed she would live to get to the hospital. She said she knew the family did not expect her to live but was surprised that he believed the same and of course she would live because she "had three children at home and had to make sure they graduated from high school." My mother had a strong faith in God and always had future oriented projects to accomplish.

Then and Now

Not much has changed over these sixty plus years. Cancer is still a frightening diagnosis, the numbers of people diagnosed with cancer is still very high, and traditional treatment remains invasive, destroys parts of the body, and suppresses the immune system. The patient continues to be very sick during treatment and for some time after if he/she survives.

My Experience with Lung Cancer

Remembering how my mother suffered from cancer and the treatment, I looked for a different way to deal with it when I was diagnosed with lung cancer in 1974. Through my prayers and meditation, and with the help of a dear friend in my "Search for God" group, I was lead to a physician who used alternative treatments that were not only successful but also non-invasive and non-debilitating, and did not destroy healthy cells in my body nor suppress the immune system. During treatment I continued teaching nursing and health students, writing articles, carrying out research and all of my usual activities with no side effects from the treatment. It was a different experience from that of my mother, friends and colleagues who elected traditional therapy.

I also remembered my mother's faith and optimism and believing it was an important part of her survival; I wanted to incorporate this into my treatment plan. Consequently I used a holistic approach that involved implementing a combination of physical, mental and spiritual activities into my daily life. Continuing this approach to life, I am now age 79 and have no chronic health problems or prescribed medications, so I have first-hand experience that this approach works with cancer and also with preventing a recurrence.

A Positive Outcome of the Cancer Experience

A couple months ago I spoke with the friend who was my major support system during my experience with cancer. She asked, "Why do you think you had cancer?" Without hesitation I answered, "In order to now offer help and encouragement to others faced with the same diagnoses." She agreed that this was also what she believed. This book is an attempt to provide encouragement and help to others who want to deal with cancer in a less invasive, less debilitating way and to help them survive and remain free of chronic illnesses and prescribed medications afterwards.

In order to better accomplish this goal I have obtained the assistance of some of the best practitioners in the field of alternative and complementary care for cancer patients. Dr. Bernie Siegel who is world famous for his practice, lecturing, and writing in cancer and mind-body medicine contributed a chapter on mind-body medicine. Dr. Francisco Contreras, Medical Director of the Oasis of Hope and one of the most famous doctors in alternative cancer treatment, contributed a chapter on lung cancer treatment based upon data from the treatment of over 120,000 cancer patients at his facility and research on the best treatments found for lung cancer. Dr. James Forsythe who is both a medical doctor and doctor of homeopathy and Medical Director of the Cancer Treatment and Screening Center of Nevada and the Center Wellness Clinic that are both in Reno, Nevada, also wrote a chapter of medical aspects of lung cancer. Dr. Forsythe is one of the three doctors interviewed about alternative treatment for cancer in Suzanne Somers' book *Knockout: Interviews with Doctors Who Are Curing Cancer*. In her book she calls him the Renaissance Man in the area of cancer treatment and he was called the "best complementary and alternative physician in the US" by Burton Goldberg – the voice of alternative medicine. Both Dr. Contreras and Dr. Forsythe can document much higher survival rates for lung cancer that those obtained by others who are using traditional treatment. Dr. Forsythe is also author of *Anti-Aging Cures: Life Changing Secrets to Reverse the Effects of Aging* with a foreword by Suzanne Somers that is available for purchase in December, 2011.

Dr. Kim Dalzell, a nationally recognized expert on oncology nutrition, has a popular book on nutrition and cancer titled *Challenge Cancer and Win!* and contributed a chapter on nutrition and lung cancer for this book. Mrs. Tanya Harter Pierce, who is author of the very popular book, *Outsmart Your Cancer: Alternative Non-Toxic Treatments That Work* which is now in its second edition, is recognized nationally as the authority on Protocel®, one of the treatments discussed in detail in her book and in this book. On August 20, 2011 Mrs. Pierce's book was ranked 6,521 of all books on Amazon, 19 in the Mind-Body category and 46 in the Alternative Health category.

Using Supplemental Holistic Interventions

Another goal for this book is to provide information to readers on how to carry out some of the supplemental holistic interventions mentioned in this book that might not be familiar to the reader. These holistic interventions discussed under the categories of physical, mental and spiritual include how to meditate, use affirmations, quit smoking, detect and remove radon from your home, and many others that relate to a holistic approach to lung cancer interventions.

Questions the Reader May Ask about Alternative Treatments

The reader may ask, "Why a book on alternative treatments for lung cancer?" First, lung cancer is the second most prevalent cancer among men and women in the United States and the leading cause of deaths from cancer. Next, the newly diagnosed patient may want to know the difference between how patients feel when being treated with traditional or with alternative treatments. Those receiving traditional treatment may experience nausea, vomiting, hair loss, fatigue, gastrointestinal upset and many other symptoms, whereas those receiving alternative treatments are usually void of these and other debilitating symptoms. Next, the patient may want to consider the success rate of these two approaches. The best estimates for patients with stage IV lung cancers are 2% chance of long-term survival with traditional therapy although those without metastasis will fair better. In contrast, physicians providing alternative treatments including those involved in this book are experiencing up to 39% survival of stage IV lung cancer patients and higher for cancers of other sites.

The reader may then question, "If alternative and complementary treatment for lung cancer is so successful and free of debilitating effects why are doctors not providing this care and why are there so few books on alternative care for lung cancer to inform the public of this option. The politics of this multi-billion dollar industry is discussed in this book and may be an eye opener for the uninformed. It should answer these two questions.

Again, my purpose is to make you, the reader, aware of the opportunities available for successful non-debilitating treatment of lung cancer and the ways to prevent a recurrence and remain healthy afterwards. It is always your choice about treatment options you select when faced with a diagnosis of lung cancer and having the information available is important for that decision-making. If I can be of any assistance, please, email me at carlhelvie@cox.net. If you want more information on natural, non-invasive interventions for any type of cancer or any of the common chronic health concerns please visit my website at www.holistichealthshow.com and listen to interviews with many of the authorities in alternative, complementary medicine and health.

Carl O. Helvie

Part I

Overview of Lung Cancer

Chapter I

Lung Cancer Overview: Types, Classification, Scope, Demographics, Etiology, Prevention, Politics, and Societal Responses to Alternative Treatments

Introduction

Cancer is the second leading cause of all deaths in the United States and lung cancer is the leading cause of cancer deaths worldwide. In addition, over half of all people diagnosed with lung cancer die within one year of their diagnoses and 75% die within two years. Thus, the current system of diagnosing and treating lung cancer is failing the public.

I am a registered nurse with a doctorate in public health and wellness who has helped many of those needing my services for 58 years as a nurse practitioner, educator, author, and researcher. I am also a 38 -year lung cancer survivor who used holistic natural alternative treatments when given 6 months to live by my physicians. This book is my contribution to others who are diagnosed with lung cancer and who want to try something different than the usual surgery, chemotherapy, and radiation that have such poor outcomes and are often disabling to the patient.

In this chapter you will read about types of lung cancer, the incidence, demographics and trends, causes and what you can do to prevent it, classification of lung cancers, a history on societal reluctance to utilize natural alternative treatments, the politics of cancer, and the current movement away from traditional and toward alternative/integrative holistic treatment of lung cancer.

Definition and Types of Lung Cancer

Definition

When cells in a part of the body grow out of control the individual is said to have cancer. Cancer is a group of diseases in which there is abnormal and unrestricted cell division and a spread of those cells into healthy tissues.

Types of Tumors (Cancerous and Non-Cancerous) in the Lungs

There are two types of lung cancer: **Non-Small Cell Lung Cancer (NSCLC)** and **Small Cell Lung Cancer (SCLC).** About 85% to 90% of all lung cancers are non-small cell cancers and are divided into three subcategories depending upon the size, shape, and chemical composition of the cells. These subcategories are squamous cell carcinoma, adenocarcinoma, and large cell undifferentiated carcinoma. Squamous cell carcinoma is responsible for 25% to 30% of all lung cancer and is usually found near the central area of the lung near the bronchi and are most often related to a history of smoking.

Adenocarcinoma is responsible for about 40% of all lung cancers and is usually found in the outer region of the lungs. Large cell undifferentiated carcinoma is responsible for about 10% to 15% of all lung cancer and may occur in any area of the lung but grows rapidly and spreads quickly resulting in a poor prognosis.

About 10% to 15% of all lung cancer is small cell cancer that tends to spread widely throughout the body. It often starts in the bronchi near the center of the chest and can multiply quickly, form large tumors and spread to the lymph nodes and other organs such as the bones, brain and liver.

In addition to the Non-Small Cell Lung Cancer and Small Cell Lung Cancer there are **non cancerous (benign) tumors** such as: 1) carcinoid tumors that are responsible for less than 5% of lung tumors and are slow growing, and 2) atypical carcinoid tumors that are rare and grow and spread rapidly. There are also **lung tumors that have spread to the lungs from other sites** such as the breast, kidneys or skin and are known as metastatic cancer.

Classification System of Lung Cancers

Non-Small Cell Lung Cancer

The system used to describe the growth and spread of NSCLC is the American Joint Committee on Cancer Staging System where T stands for Tumor and includes its size and the distance it has spread within the lung and nearby organs, N signifies its spread to lymph nodes and M signifies it has metastasized or spread to distance organs. These three factors (tumor, nodes, and metastasis) are combined and a stage is assigned to each specific grouping as follows.

T Categories (size and location):

Tis. Cancer in the layer of cells lining the air passage but has not invaded other lung tissue.

T1. Cancer 3 cm (just under 1¼ inch) or less and has not spread to the membranes surrounding the lung nor the main branch of the bronchi.

T2. Cancer includes one or more of the following characteristics:

- larger than 3 cm
- involves a main bronchus 2 cm (about ¾ inch) or more from the point where the trachea (windpipe) branches into the left and right main bronchi (carina).
- involves the membranes surrounding the lungs (pleura)
- may partially clog the airways but not to the extent of causing the lung to collapse or to develop pneumonia.

T3. Cancer includes one of more of the following:

- spread to any of the following: chest wall, the diaphragm (breathing muscle separating the chest from the abdomen), mediastinal pleura (membrane between the two lungs), or parietal pericardium (membrane of sac surrounding the heart)

- invades a main bronchus closer than 2 cm (about ¾ inch) to the point where the trachea branches into the right and left main bronchi but does not affect it
- airways affected to the point where an entire lung has collapsed or there is pneumonia in a lung.

T4. Cancer includes one or more of the following:

- invaded the mediastinum (space behind chest bone and in front of the heart), trachea (windpipe), esophagus (tube connecting the throat and stomach), the backbone, or carina (point where wind pipe branches into left and right main bronchi)
- two or more separate tumor nodules found in the same lobe
- a malignant pleural effusion is present (fluid containing cancer cells surrounding the lung).

N Categories (lymph nodes near lungs affected):

N0. No spread to lymph nodes.

N1. Lymph nodes within the lung and/or around the area where the bronchus enters the lung are affected, and nodes are only on the side of the cancerous lung.

N2. Lymph nodes in the area where the trachea branches into the left and right bronchi or in the space behind the chest bone and in front of the heart are affected. The affected lymph nodes are on the same side as the cancerous lung.

N3. Lymph nodes are near the collarbone on either side or hilar or mediastinal lymph nodes on the opposite side of the cancerous lung are involved.

M Categories (Metastasis or where the cancer has spread):

M0. No spread to distance organs or areas (other lobes of the lung, lymph nodes beyond those identified in N stages or other organs such as bone, brain or liver).

M1. Cancer spread to one or more distant sites (the other lung, a different lobe of the same lung, another organ, or a second tumor in a different part of the lung but independent of the first).

Staging of Groups

Grouping the TNM information allows for a stage category that identifies tumor types that have a similar prognosis and are thus treated in a similar way. Stages include 0, I, II, III, and IV in which those with a lower stage number have a better prognosis.

Stage 0. Tis, N0, M0

Cancer has invaded only the layer of cells lining the air passage but has not moved to other lung tissue or spread to lymph nodes or distant sites.

Stage I A. T1, N0, M0

Cancer size is less than 3 cm, has not spread to membranes surrounding the lungs, does not affect the main branches of the bronchi, and has not spread to lymph nodes or distant sites.

Stage I B. T2, N0, M0

Cancer is larger than 3 cm, or involves a main bronchus but is not near the carina, or has spread to the pleura, or is partially clogging the airway. It has not spread to the lymph nodes or distant sites.

Stage II A. T1, N1, M0

Cancer is 3 cm or less, has not spread to the membranes surrounding the lungs, and does not affect the main branch of the bronchi. It has spread to nearby or hilar lymph nodes but has not spread to distant sites.

Stage II B. T2, N1, M0, or T3, N0, M0

Cancer is over 3 cm, or involves a main bronchus but is not near the carina, or has spread to the pleura, or is partially clogging the airway. It has spread to nearby or hilar lymph nodes but not to distant sites, or it has spread to the chest wall or the diaphragm, the mediastinal pleura, or membranes surrounding the heart, or it spread to a main bronchus and is close to the carina, or it has grown into the airways enough to cause an entire lung to collapse or to cause pneumonia in the entire lung. It has not spread to lymph nodes or distant sites.

Stage III A. T1 or 2, N2, M0 or T3, N1, or 2, M0

Cancer can be any size, involves a main bronchus but is not near the carina, or it has spread to the pleura, or is partially clogging an airway. It has spread to mediastinum nodes (middle of the chest), but not to distant sites, or it has spread to chest wall or the diaphragm, the mediastinal pleura, or membranes surrounding the heart, or it invades a main bronchus and is close to the carina, or it has grown into the airway causing an entire lung to collapse or pneumonia in the entire lung. It has spread to lymph nodes anywhere in the chest on the same side as the cancer but not to distant sites.

Stage III B. T1, 2, or 3, N3, M 0, or T4, any N, M0

Cancer is any size and has spread to the lymph nodes around the collar bone on either side or hilar or mediastinal lymph nodes on the opposite side of the cancerous lung, or it has spread to the mediastinum, heart, trachea, esophagus, backbone, or the carina, or two or more separate tumor nodules are present in the same lobe, or there is fluid containing cancer cells in the area surrounding the lung. The cancer may or may not have spread to lymph nodes and has not spread to distant sites.

Stage IV. Any T, Any N, M1

Cancer has spread to distant sites.

Staging of Small Cell Lung Cancer

Unlike other types of cancer that use a 4-stage system, a two-stage system is used for small cell lung cancer. This system classifies limited and extensive stages where limited means the cancer is only in one lung and in the lymph nodes on the same side of the chest. Extensive stage is used for small cell lung cancers that have spread to the other lung, to lymph nodes on the other side of the chest, or to distant organs. This system separates those patients who have a fair prognosis with treatment from those who have a worse outlook with little chance of cure.

Scope of Lung Cancer in the United States and Worldwide: Incidence, Mortality and Survival Rates
US Mortality (Death) Rates

Cancer is the second leading cause of death in the United States. One out of every 4 individuals and 3 out of 4 families will be affected by cancer at some time. The largest number of cancer cases is found in four areas of the body: lungs, colon-rectum, breast, and prostate.

We often hear and read about breast and prostate cancers in the media but less about lung cancer. Consequently, you may ask, "Why a book on lung cancer?" Would you be surprised to hear that lung cancer is the most common cause of death due to cancer in men and women worldwide and that in the United States the death rate for lung cancer in women is higher than for breast cancer? Further, according to the American Cancer Society (2007), in 2005 lung cancer killed more people in the United States that the total deaths from breast, prostate and colon cancers. In 2008 there were an estimated 161,840 deaths from lung cancer in the United States (Jemal et al, 2009). Thus, it is a major health concern.

US Incidence Rates (New Cases)

How common is lung cancer in the United States? It is the second most common cancer among both men and women. The National Cancer Institute (NCI, 2007) estimated that approximately one out of every 4 men and women would be diagnosed with lung cancer at some time during their lifetime. In 2008 there were 215,020 estimated new lung cancer cases in the United States (Jemal et al, 2009). The American Cancer Society (2007) estimates that there will be 219,440 new cases and 159,390 deaths from lung cancer in 2009.

Worldwide Statistics

In 2002 there were 10.9 million new cases, 6.7 million deaths, and 24.6 million people alive with all types of cancer within three years of diagnosis worldwide. The most common diagnosed cancer worldwide was lung cancer (1.35 million) and the most common cause of death from cancer was lung cancer (1.18 million). These figures vary by country from an age specific incidence rate of under 10 per 100,000 people in parts of China, Africa, and South America to over 100 in some Black populations in the United States. The most prevalent (old and new cases per 100,000 population) cancer worldwide was breast cancer (4.4 million survivors up to 5 years after diagnoses) (Parkin, DM et al, 2005)

Lung Cancer Survival

The previously quoted statistics show that lung cancer patients usually do not live long after being diagnosed. Survival rates for NSCLC survivors for 1992-93 were: Stage I–47%, Stage II–26%, Stage III–8%, and Stage IV–2% (American Cancer Society, 2007). The relative 5-year survival rates for SCLC is around 21% if found early and is localized within the lung without any spread to lymph nodes. This category comprises about 6% of all small cell cancer patients. If there is any sign of spread the small cells relative 5-year survival rate is about 11% and that accounts for about 34% of the small cell cancer patients. If there is extensive disease the survival rate is 2%. An overall 5-year lung cancer survival rate following diagnosis in the United States for all stages is 14% according to Al-Kayer (2006).

Gender, Racial and Age Distribution of Lung Cancer
Gender

The statistics for gender distribution of lung cancer show the rate for men is higher than for women in each racial group. It was estimated that in 2008 there would be 114,690 new lung cancer cases among men in the United States and 90,810 deaths. Among women in the United States 100,330 new cases of lung cancer were estimated for 2008 and 71,030 deaths.

Racial Distribution

Racial distribution of lung cancer show an age adjusted *incidence* rate (new cases per 100,000) among men that range from a low of 14 among American Indians to a high of 117 among blacks, an eight-fold difference. Between these extremes there are two categories ranging from 42 to 53 for Hispanics, Japanese, Chinese, Filipinos, and Koreans and from 71 to 89 for Vietnamese, Caucasians, Alaska Natives and Hawaiians. The age-adjusted *mortality* (death) rates follow a similar pattern as those for incidence. Among men, the mortality (death rate) and incidence rates (new cases) are very similar except for Filipino men who have an incidence rate almost twice that of the mortality rate.

The incidence rate for women range from 15 per 100,000 among Japanese women to almost 51 among Alaskan natives. Between these extremes a group of 16 and 25 cases per 100,000 includes Koreans, Filipinos, Hispanics, and Chinese women, and a group between 31 and 44 cases includes Vietnamese, Caucasian women, Hawaiian and Black women. Mortality rates among women are similar to incidence rates except for Filipino and Hispanic women. Their incidence rates are nearly twice as large as their mortality rates possibly due to recording errors.

Age Distribution

Al-Kayer (2006) says the incidence of lung cancer rises sharply with age. Lung cancer is predominately a disease of the elderly and almost 70% of all new cases are over 65 years of age. A breakdown by age shows: almost 53% of all new cases in the United States are over 70; almost 27% are between 60 and 69; almost 15% are between age 50 and 59; and almost 6% are under age 50.

Trends

Cancer was uncommon prior to the 1930s but increased dramatically over the following decades. In his video, Mazzucco (2010) dramatizes trends of cancer by saying at the beginning of the 20th century there was 1 case of cancer for every 20 people over a person's lifetime. In the 1940s this rose to 1 in 16, in the 1970s it rose to 1 in 10 and today it is 1 in 3 people.

Lung cancer has been the most prevalent cancer worldwide since 1985 and by 2002 there were 1.35 million new cases that represented 12.4% of all new cancer cases. Lung cancer was also the most common cause of deaths from cancer with 1.18 million deaths, or 17.6% of the total cancer deaths worldwide in 2002. Overall, the cancer rate has decreased very little over time. For example, the *New York Times* stated that after adjusting for the size and age of the population, cancer mortality dropped only 5% over the 55 years from 1950 to 2005. However, according to Jemal, et al (2009) the incidence rate has recently started to decline. He says, "Lung cancer incidence rates are declining in men and plateauing in women after increasing for many years."

Causes of Lung Cancer

Risk factors for lung cancer include cigarette smoking and second-hand smoke, exposure to selected industrial chemicals such as asbestos and arsenic; exposure to radiation including radon, and the use of selected immunoenhancing foods. Each of these will be discussed briefly below.

A Word about Multi-causal Lung Cancer Process

A word is in order about adhering too closely to causal factors for lung cancer because it is known that not everyone who smokes gets lung cancer and some who do not smoke will get it. This is true for each of the causal factors identified above. Instead of a single cause there are multiple factors that determine diseases and health in humans and these involve variations in humans, in the disease, injury producing or health agent, and in the environment that brings them together. Health or illness result when there is the right combination of these factors. For example, lung cancer host factors might include age (most lung cancer is in the 65 year old and older), health condition, attitudes and emotions (research shows that optimism increases a positive outcome for lung cancer), habits, and others whereas environ-mental factors could include nutrition available and used (green leafy vegetables have been shown to prevent cancer in smokers and soy products may decrease lung cancer risk if smoking is stopped), supplements taken (vitamin B6 has a protective effect on lung cancer and vitamin B17 has been used successfully in prevention and treatment) stress in the work or social environment, other smokers in the social environment, and agent factors (the cigarettes or cigars) might include different brands with different amounts of tar and nicotine. For lung cancer to occur the person is most often older and has been a heavy smoker for a number of years, is negative about his life situation and often feels stressed, who eats junk food most of the time, combined with an environment that places demand beyond the person's coping ability, and who associates with other heavy smokers, and who smokes a cigarette that is high in tar, nicotine and chemicals. Although this is a hypothetical example, epidemi-ological research data is used to piece together the causal factors of all health and disease processes. This framework is useful for health interventions because if health and illness are processes it is possible to intervene at various levels in the process to change an illness process into a healthy one. For example, a person who quits smoking early in the process, starts eating a better nutritional diet, and finds a less stressful job will decrease his risk for lung cancer. This is a simplified overview of the public health process used to keep the public healthy and puts the causation of lung cancer into perspective. The interested reader is referred to some of the author's earlier books where he put together a framework based upon multiple concepts to explain preventive care in the community (Helvie, 1998, 1991). Although different concepts may be used, this framework is also useful to view holistic health care that is the model used for interventions in my own life during and after treatment for lung cancer. With these concepts in mind the reader is now offered the most likely causes for lung cancer in populations.

Tobacco Smoking

The major cause of lung cancer is tobacco smoking (cigarette, pipe, and cigar) accounting for more than 87% of all cases. Data from 1979 reported that 90% of the lung cancer deaths in males and 79% in females were due to cigarette smoking (Blot et all, 1996).

There are additional cases among non-smokers who develop it from environmental passive exposure to smoke that account for around 3% of all cases. Smoking more than 20 cigarettes a day confers a risk of between 15- and 25-fold relative to nonsmokers (Hammond, EC, 1966; Doll, R et al, 1995; and McLaughlin et al, 1995). In addition, the risk of developing lung cancer for a non-smoker living with a smoker is 30% greater than a non-smoker living with a non-smoking partner and one hour of secondary smoke is equal to smoking 4 cigarettes. The longer you smoke and the more you smoke each day increases the risk of developing lung cancer. If you stop smoking before a tumor develops you reduce your risk and by 10 years this reduction is 1/3 of what it would have been had you continued smoking. A study in 2010 found that **early** lung cancer smokers who quit can double their survival chances. In the study those who did not quit had a 29% to 33% survival in 5 years whereas those who quit had a 63% to 70% survival. Research in 2010 also showed that a diet including ample green leafy vegetables might offer protection among smokers against lung cancer.

Cigar and pipe smoking are almost as likely to cause lung cancer as cigarette smoking. In addition, there is no evidence that low tar cigarettes reduce the risk of lung cancer.

Asbestos

Those working with asbestos in the workplace are 7 times more likely to die of lung cancer and those who also smoke have a 50 to 70 times greater risk than people in general. Asbestos as a risk factor has been reduced in recent years because of governmental regulations that ended the use of asbestos in residential and commercial products. Although it is still present in many older homes and businesses it is not considered dangerous as long as it is not released into the air by demolition or renovation.

There are 5,000 deaths in the US annually related to asbestos.

Arsenic

Arsenic is a well-documented human carcinogen and lung cancer has been associated with chronic arsenic exposure in smelter and pesticide workers. A higher risk of lung cancer was found among workers exposed predominantly to arsenic trioxide in smelters and to pentavalent arsenical pesticides in other settings (ATSDR, 2007).

Chronic inhalation of arsenicals has been associated with lung cancer (Falk et al, 1981). According to IARC and NRC, the association between chronic arsenic exposure and cancer is strongest for skin, lung, and bladder cancer. Liver (angiosarcoma), kidney, and other cancers have limited strength of association (IARC, 2004; NRC, 2000). The association between lung cancer and occupational exposure to inorganic arsenic has been confirmed in several epidemiological studies (Enterline et al, 1987), and arsenic is considered a cause of lung as well as skin cancer. In his review he found: 1) in arsenic-exposed workers, there is a systematic gradient in lung cancer mortality rates, depending upon duration and intensity of exposure (ATSDR, 2007); and 2) neither concomitant exposure to sulfur dioxide nor to cigarette smoke was determined to be an essential co-factor in these studies

A study published in 2004 (How-Ran Guo et al) also looked at lung cancer and arsenic. The study included 243 townships in Taiwan. Patients were identified through the National Cancer Registry and lung cancer patients in 5 epidemic areas with arsenic in the drinking water were compared with 238 other townships. To control for age and gender the subjects were divided into male and female, and into 4 age groups. There were 37,290 lung cancer patients (26,850 men and 10,440 women) diagnosed between January 1, 1980 and December 31, 1999. Patients from the high epidemic arsenic areas had high rates of squamous cell and small cell carcinomas, but lower rates of adenocarcinomas and these results were similar across all age groups. Data on smoking history was not available. The researchers concluded that the carconogenicity of arsenic on lungs is cell specific related to arsenic ingestion and suggest that arsenic may have different mechanisms in the development of lung cancer through exposure via different routes (drinking vs inhalation).

In a study by Yu-tang and Zhen (1996) the incidence of lung cancer for workers who had been exposed to insoluble arsenic in four mines was found to be $290/10^5$. In another study reported in the UC Newsroom (2010) the researchers found that the death rates for those exposed to arsenic continued to be high as long as

20 years after exposure. For men the rate of lung and bladder cancer was 152 deaths per 100,000 population and for women it was 50 per 100,000. This was 2½ to 3 times higher than in areas without arsenic in the water.

Radon

Radon is a radioactive gas that cannot be seen, tasted or smelled and that results from the natural breakdown of uranium. It may be in the earth under a home and seep into your living spaces creating a concentration of the gas that may cause lung cancer. Living in a home that is contaminated may increase your risk of lung cancer by 2 or 3 times. The risk is increased for smokers. Radon, found in many homes, accounts for an estimated 5,000 to 20,000 deaths in the US annually (Koren, 1991) and is the second leading cause of lung cancer (Murdock, 1991).

Other Pollutants

Power plants pollute the environment and a 2004 report (Clear the Air) says it is responsible for: 1) 24,000 American lives annually with 2,800 of those from lung cancer; and 2) 38,200 non-fatal heart attacks annually. It was also responsible for 21,850 hospital admissions; 26,000 emergency room visits for asthma; 16,200 chronic bronchitis attacks; 554,000 asthma attacks; and 3,186,000 lost days from work. Power plants were also responsible for 474 counties in the US failing to meet minimum air pollution health standards according to the Environmental Protection Agency and reported in Clean the Air (2004).

Diets Low in Fruit and Vegetables

A diet low in fruit and vegetables has also been identified as a causal factor for lung cancer. When I had lung cancer in 1974 my diet was 75% raw fruit and vegetables and protein was prohibited. Currently there is more emphasis on research of specific aspects of fruit and vegetables as they relate to lung cancer. A recent study reported that green leafy vegetables protect against lung cancer even in smokers. Another study found that soy products reduce the risk of lung cancer. Nutrition including fruit and vegetables is so important in the prevention and treatment of lung cancer that a chapter is devoted to this subject later in this book.

Prevention of Lung Cancer

The risk for lung cancer can be reversed if the individual knows what the risk factors are and makes the decision to change his/her behavior and changes the risky behavior. Reducing the risk of lung cancer includes smoking cessation, avoidance of secondary smoke in restaurants, public and private buildings and at home; wearing appropriate clothing and using proper equipment while working with industrial chemicals such as asbestos; assessing for radon levels and making necessary changes in the home; reducing exposure to x-rays in doctors' offices and to ultraviolet radiation in direct sunlight, and replacing immune-suppressing foods (processed foods, sugar) with immune-enhancing ones such as fresh fruits and vegetables, whole grains, and flax oil. These and other holistic interventions will be discussed in Chapters 9 and 10 where the specifics of smoking cessation, radon detection and removal from the home, and other interventions are elaborated.

Traditional vs. Integrative Interventions for Lung Cancer

A comparison of the side effects and survival outcomes of traditional and integrative interventions for lung cancer will show that integrative interventions are more natural, non-invasive and usually without or with minimal side effects. In addition, the 5-year survival for patients receiving integrative interventions is much higher than for those receiving traditional treatments. Some of these comparisons are presented in the next section. After reading these, you may ask, "If patients receiving integrative interventions have limited or no side effects and have a much higher probability of survival than those receiving traditional treatment why does surgery, chemotherapy and radiation continue as the treatment of choice?" Although this is a complex subject, some of the factors involved in this answer will now be discussed.

Discouraging Integrative or Alternative Cancer Treatment
Laetrile (Vitamin B17)

There has been a concerted effort on the part of the FDA and Drug Companies to suppress alternative treatments that will not give them a profit. In my own life, I have found this to be true with laetrile that was the treatment I selected (see Chapter 2) after I was diagnosed with lung cancer 38 years ago. At that time I found a physician in Virginia who would treat me using laetrile. He had worked for the National Cancer Institute providing successful cancer treatment and carrying out research with laetrile but was reportedly closed down by the FDA and Drug Companies. Because of his success with this cancer intervention, he continued providing treatment under the table, so to speak, so I was asked to sign papers that I would not report him or sue him. At that time, I could easily find apricot kernels, the highest source of laetrile, in most health food stores and used these to supplement the laetrile. My doctor also told me where I could obtain laetrile. Over the years it became almost impossible to find these in any health food store and only occasionally on the Internet. A check on the Internet a few years ago showed that both my physician's office and the pharmacy where I purchased the laetrile had been closed. More recently I found apricot kernels and laetrile locally and on the Internet but suspect these sources will disappear when discovered.

Despite convincing evidence that laetrile was and is extremely effective in the treatment of cancer every physician who successfully treated cancer patients in the United States was harassed and often required to defend himself at great expense. The success of laetrile in cancer treatment and the harassment of physicians who used it is well documented in *World Without Cancer* (Griffin, 2009), *Outsmart Your Cancer* (Harter-Pierce, 2009), and *Cancer: The Forbidden Cures* (Mazzucco, 2010). Some courageous physicians who are more committed to the recovery of their patients than a large bank account continue to use laetrile successfully today in the United States, Mexico, and Europe.

In addition, current traditional books on cancer that mention laetrile label it as quackery and state that it contains cyanide and will kill you. I guess because I didn't know this when I took it and also ate apricot kernels daily for 2 years it did not affect me.

For example, in their book, *Definitive Guide to Cancer*, Alschuler and Gazella (2007) state, "Laetrile ingested in the form of apricot kernels or administered intravenously can be linked to cyanide toxicity in susceptible individuals, can cause severe heart rate disturbances, breathing problems, and coma. Treatment usually requires intensive care hospitalization. Taking laetrile along with conventional treatment can increase the potential for cyanide poisoning. Laetrile is **illegal** in the United States." Although I know and have respect for one of the authors and find her extremely knowledgeable about many types of complementary and alternative treatments for cancer as taught in naturopathic school, I find this information incorrect and frightening for the uninformed reader. If you believed this to be true would you take laetrile? No, I would not either. In truth, there are small amounts of cyanide in the apricot kernels (a natural product) and in laetrile that acts on the tumor ONLY but not on the normal tissue. This process is discussed in Chapter 2. Thus, the cyanide in laetrile kills the cancer cells but does not affect healthy cells.

I have never heard of or read case studies involving the severe consequences discussed above. In addition, Dr. Contreras, Medical Director of the Oasis of Hope, where over 100,000 cancer patients from 55 countries have been treated and who wrote Chapter 4 in this book, told me that they have discovered from their research of treatments for lung cancer that laetrile is one of the effective treatments currently available for lung cancer. In addition, laetrile treatment is currently **legal** in at least 3 of the 50 states in the United States according to Dr. Robert Eslinger of the Reno Integrative Clinic and other alternative physicians. These states are Nevada, Arizona and Connecticut and require additional study and certification of the physician who practices integrative treatment of cancer.

In the literature you will find positive comments about laetrile going back many years. For example, a letter from Dr. Dean Burk (Griffin, 2009) stated: "With forty-five years of study and research on the cancer problem, the last thirty-three years in the US National Cancer Institute, and with files of virtually all published literature on the use of amygdalin ('laetrile') with reference to cancer, and with innumerable files of unpublished documents and letters, I have found no statements of demonstrated pharmacological harmfulness of amygdalin to human beings at any dosage recommended or employed by medical doctors in the United States and abroad." A second comment by Dr. DM Greenberg, Professor Emeritus of Bio-Chemistry at the University of California at Berkeley and consultant to the Cancer Advisory council in California stated: "There is no question that pure amygdalin (laetrile) is a non-toxic compound. This is not questioned by anyone who has studied the reports submitted to the Cancer Advisory Council of the State of California" (Griffin, 2009, 102). The interested reader is referred to Griffin's book that is both comprehensive and well documented.

On the other hand consider the effect of the traditional 3 treatments for cancer on the individual. Chemotherapy, a drug and one of the traditional treatments of choice, has severe side effects such as nausea and vomiting, hair loss, mouth sores, dry mouth, diarrhea or constipation, fatigue, dental problems, loss of appetite, taste impairment, anemia, infections, cardiovascular damage, and neuropathy according to most scientific literature. Likewise, all chemicals have harmful side effects and even "aspirin tablets are twenty times more toxic than the equivalent amount of laetrile. Each year in the United States, over ninety people die of aspirin poisoning. No one ever has died of B17" (Griffin, 2009, 102). "It is estimated that 100,000 people die every year from prescription drugs" (Griffin, 2009, 103). Barry (2011) says according to a recent study by the federal Agency for Healthcare Research and Quality "adverse drug effects send about 4.5 million Americans to the doctor's office or the emergency room each year…" and "estimates that serious drug reactions occur more that 2 million times each year in hospitals and are the fourth leading cause of hospital deaths." She further states that these serious and fatal reactions reported are only the tip of the iceberg according to experts.

Radiation, a second traditional choice treatment, may cause anemia, fatigue, nausea and vomiting, sterility, skin burns, hair loss, diarrhea, fatigue. Surgery, the third treatment of choice, is invasive and always carries the danger of such conditions as MRSA and other infections. Recently a friend, who had anesthesia during surgery for breast cancer, had an onset of Alzheimer's shortly thereafter. Although it did not cause the problem, the doctor told the family that it hastened the condition that was previously hidden.

In addition, the survival rates of those receiving traditional treatments for lung cancer are poor (see information on survival rates earlier in this chapter). Survival rates obtained by specific leaders in integrative cancer treatment in the US and Mexico are consistently higher. For example, Dr. Contreras at the Oasis of Hope evaluates survival rates of patients with stage IV lung, breast, colorectal, and ovarian cancer they have treated using integrative interventions and says, "Oasis of Hope patients are doing considerably better than those receiving integrative cancer treatment at Cancer Treatment Centers of America and/or the average standard of care in the US. In fact, 5-year cancer survival in each of these cancers is at least 2–3-fold higher than in patients receiving conventional cancer therapy – in some cases, greater." Tables on his website show that for lung cancer the Oasis of Hope has a 62% higher survival after 1 year, 44% higher survival after 2 years and 7.4% higher survival after 5 years. More information is available at: http://www.oasisofhope.com/patient-survival-statistics.php. Dr. James Forsythe in Nevada refers to survival rates for his clients and says, "At five years out, our response rate is much better than conventional chemotherapy, which is at 2%. We are getting 35 to 40% survivorship and these are all stage IV cancers. The excellent response does not carry with it any adverse side effects" (Somers, 2009, 124). In a later cohort of survivors he received even higher rates. Other success rates are identified below for specific integrative treatments.

There have also been efforts on the part of the government and drug companies to discourage integrative physicians from using successful non-debilitating natural treatments with cancer patients. A few of these will be mentioned below and further information can be found in *Outsmart Your Cancer* (Pierce, 2009) and a new DVD titled *Cancer: The Forbidden Cures* (Mazzucco, 2010).

Hoxsey Formula
Harry Hoxsey was another who received a negative response from the drug companies, FDA, and medical associations. He was a naturopathic physician who specialized in cancer and became involved in a major conflict with the American medical politics because of his advocacy and use of controversial non-surgical, and non-radiological treatments. During the 1930s, 40s and 50s he and the doctors with whom he worked cured thousands of cancer patients and gained widespread publicity. In the 1950s he had the largest cancer clinic in the United States with

branch clinics in 17 states treating over 10,000 patients. The attention generated by his successes led to harassment and attempts by the medical profession and governmental agencies to destroy these and other promising cancer treatments and is well documented in two books (Hoxsey, 1956; Ausubel, 2000). Despite an 80% success rate with his cancer treatment he was arrested around 100 times in two years in Texas. He was always out of jail in a day or two and carried $100 bills in his pocket for this purpose. The DA could never persuade any of his patients to testify against him and when the DA's own brother secretly used the Hoxsey formula and his cancer disappeared, the DA became one of Hoxsey's lawyers and one of his best advocates. At one point in his career he was approached by and refused to give exclusive rights for his treatments to the president of the American Medical Association and a group of their doctors. Thereafter, they began harassing him and calling him a quack. Hoxsey sued the American Medical Association for libel and slander and the case went as high as the Supreme Court where he won. However, immediately thereafter the FDA padlocked all 176 of his clinics for using unapproved medicine.

Hoxsey was successfully defended after each attack. In fact, on one occasion in 1954, a group of 10 doctors from around the United States independently investigated Hoxsey's clinic in Dallas. They examined case histories, and talked with patients and ex-patients. They reported that the clinic was successfully treating pathologically proven cases of cancer without the use of surgery, radium or x-ray and that the Hoxsey treatments were superior to conventional methods of treatment and they were willing to assist in any way possible to bring his treatment to the American public. However, the continual harassment by the medical association and the Federal Drug Administration drove Hoxsey's clinic to Mexico. Interestingly, even Hoxsey's nurse, Mildred Nelson, joined his staff in 1946 to expose him as a hoax. After her mother was successfully treated by him for cancer and she saw many successes from his treatments she became a strong advocate of his work, became the director in 1963 and remained until her passing in 1999.

Essiac Tea

Renee Caisse was a Canadian public health nurse who searched for a cancer cure in the 1920s when her aunt contracted terminal cancer. She found a woman who used an Indian tea and had cured herself of breast cancer. The tea (Essiac Tea) was made of burdock, sheep's sorrel, slippery elm, and Indian rhubarb root. Using this tea her aunt was cured and she named the tea after her last name spelled backwards, thus, becoming Essiac Tea. The tea was used successfully with thousands of her patients in her public health nursing practice and later in a clinic that she used from 1934 to 1942. Although there were many efforts to suppress her treatments by the Canadian government and medical profession she continued sometimes in secret and after her death her tea continued to be used successfully and continues to be used today by some cancer patients.

Other Alternative Treatments

In her book, *Outsmart Your Cancer* (2009), Tanya Harter Pierce discusses many of the other effective alternative treatments for cancer such as Burzynski's Antineoplastons, Protocel®, the Gerson Method, Dr. Kelley's Enzyme Therapy and others, and the efforts of the government and drug companies to suppress these therapies. The interested reader is referred to this reference as well as *Cancer: The Forbidden Cures* (Mazzucco, 2010) that discusses these and other treatments on a DVD. In addition, Somers (2009) discusses the treatments and success rates of some of the current practicing integrative cancer physicians. Connie Strasheim (2011) discussed 15 naturopathic and integrative doctors who discuss how they defeat cancer. Eidem (1997) discusses Dr. Emanuel Revici who successfully treated cancer and AIDS, and two additional DVD's, *Cancer is Curable Now* (Connealy, L), and *Burzynski* (Friedman, M MD) demonstrate the success of doctors treating cancer.

Suppression of Successful Alternative Treatments Continue Today
Efforts to suppress natural alternative integrative therapies and the physicians who are using them continue today. Some of the physicians discussed in Pierce's book are *currently* working in the cancer field. In addition, a search of alternative doctors and disciplinary action on Goggle or a review of Quackwatch will turn up many others whose main goal is to cure patients with natural non-invasive treatments. Some of the leaders in the field of medicine are listed on these sites and the story of Dr. Frank Shallenberger is typical. On his website http://truthaboutshallenberger.com he is supported by many of his colleagues in medicine and his story is presented. A brief summary follows: He has been in medicine for 36 years and started in emergency medicine in a shock trauma clinic which was gratifying and fulfilling because he was saving lives. After 7 years he went into private practice and saw patients with all kinds of chronic conditions such as arthritis, diabetes, hypertension and fatigue. Then he became disillusioned with conventional medicine because his patients were not getting better despite the best of modern medicine. Some actually got sicker from the drugs they were given. When he talked with colleagues about the situation they said he was doing a good job and encouraged his continuing the traditional treatments. Subsequently, he started learning alternative treatments and read about nutrition and vitamins, acupuncture, chelation therapy, oxidation therapies and others that were discussed in the literature at that early stage of alternative treatment. Because there were few studies on these treatments at that time he developed three criteria for his using a treatment: 1) safety; 2) inexpensive; and 3) some evidence that it was successful. Using these criteria he found that his patients

were getting better in "droves" and he gained a reputation of curing people who were not getting cured elsewhere. Word spread by word of mouth from patients and open-minded doctors who also started sending their most "hopeless" patients.

At this time, the State of California also began noticing and some of his colleagues began being persecuted by the bureaucracy and suffered loss of license, legal fees for defense of up to $250,000, and one friend spent more than that to defend himself for using vitamin A for a patient with an ear infection. Although the patient was happy with the treatment, his friend lost both his license and money. Of interest, the Business and Professional Code of California considered B vitamins and magnesium to be "dangerous drugs".

Knowing it was only a matter of time before they came after him, he decided to move to Nevada where there was less hostility toward alternative treatments. Following the selling of his practice, one of his former patients was hospitalized after being treated by the new owner. At about the same time, a patient submitted a claim to her insurance company for her treatment and the adjuster reported Dr. Shallenberger to the California Medical Board and found additional instances of "unacceptable" treatment. Although there was never any harm to patients he had broken the 'rules' and the board proceeded to revoke his license. The cost of fighting this would be about $200,000 and multiple trips back to California so he surrendered his California license and paid the fine.

In the foreword to *Defeat Cancer* (Strasheim, 2011) Richard Linchitz, MD says, "As I read *Defeat Cancer* I was struck by the fact that all of the doctors demonstrate incredible courage to face disapproval and, sometimes, outright attacks from mainstream medicine. In this regard, Stanislow Bursynski, MD, is almost in a class by himself. He has probably been the most persecuted and prosecuted doctor in modern history of 'alternative' medicine. He faced fourteen years of attacks by the FDA and conventional doctors, and spent millions of dollars before he finally prevailed."

Traditional Therapies for Lung and Other Cancers Driven by Politics

Concurrent with the process of discouraging alternative treatments for cancer has been a trend to perpetuate the triad of treatments (chemotherapy, surgery, radiation) based upon politics. This historical process will be discussed briefly here and is based upon the information presented in *The Politics of Cancer Therapy* (Griffin, 2009).

In a lecture on *The Politics of Cancer Therapy* Griffin using information from public records concludes that the politics of cancer treatment is more complicated than the science because there is so much money involved. His book further sets the stage by saying, "Why has orthodox medicine waged war against this non-drug (laetrile) approach?" The author contends that "the answer is to be found, not in science, but in politics – and is based upon the hidden economic and power agenda of those who dominate the medical establishment."

Griffin reviewed local, state and governmental records to collect data for his lecture so this data is available for anyone who wishes to validate the facts. He says after World War I a cartel or community of interest under IG Farben was formed for dye chemicals in Germany and later expanded to all commercial chemicals including drugs. In this cartel members agreed not to compete in order to keep prices high and this effectively did away with free enterprise where competition leads to lower prices. The cartel expanded with layering of agreements until areas of competition became narrower and the cartel extended worldwide into 93 countries. Over 2000 companies had cooperative interlocking agreements with IG Farben who dominated all of Germany and most of Europe and the United States. These include such known companies as Abbott Labs, Borden, Alcoa,

Eastman, Ford Rubber, General Motors, Nestlé, Glidden Paints, Texaco and many others. In addition, hundreds more were totally owned or controlled by IG Farben including companies such as Bayer, Lederly Labs, Roche Labs, Lesser Labs, Bristol Labs, Squibb & Sons. Thus, a pattern of cooperation was established among a large part of the organizations around the world. This prevented competition and caused a subsequent price elevation.

After World War I when Germany was defeated the industrialists believed they lost the war because they lacked gas so the top chemists at IG Farben were charged with producing gas from something abundant in Germany. These chemists developed the hydrogenation process whereby oil could be developed from coal. This allowed Germany to be self-sufficient.

The president of Standard Oil in New Jersey (a part of the Rockefeller empire) was invited by IG Farben to see the new process and to join with them in a cartel agreement of no competition for 3 years. The agreement included 3 components: 1) Standard Oil would be given ½ interest of the hydrogenation process everywhere in the world except Germany; 2) IG Farben would be given 456,000 shares of Standard Oil stock that was valued at over 30 million dollars in 1929; and 3) both agreed not to compete in the future (drugs or whatever).

During the reign of Hitler IG Farben was the money behind his rise to power in Germany and with Hitler in power it was possible to influence legislation that would insure cooperation and high prices for those who were part of the cartel. Thus, industrialists controlled the states in Germany and fair trade laws were passed that prevented shopkeepers from lowering prices. Consequently, high prices prevailed. The same happened in the United States when the FDA was established and anti-quackery laws were passed to protect consumers from health foods. This allowed the FDA and other agencies to use the anti-quackery laws to harass physicians who used natural treatments that were low cost and not controlled by the cartels. The harassment was to remove competition and keep prices high. This forced most physicians to use drugs that were controlled and expensive and make money for the drug companies and others who thrive from the hardship of cancer patients.

Following the agreement between Standard Oil and IG Farben the process of establishing cooperation to maintain high prices for drugs, and setting chemotherapy, radiation, and surgery as the traditional treatment for cancer was established. Rockefeller who had been given control of drugs in the United States established a link with cancer through tax-exempt foundations. Tax-exempt foundations allowed the family to keep their vast fortune from inheritance taxes, and use those dollars for profitable ventures. One profitable venture was cancer research. If they gave one million dollars of tax-exempt money each year for research on a couple of new toxic and expensive drugs and gave or sold these to doctors who sold them to patients, they would get their one million dollars back with several more.

Then the Rockefeller Foundations set out to take over the medical schools. The Rockefellers and Carnegies financed a report on the condition of the medical schools. For this report, known as the Flexner Report, all medical schools were surveyed and it was concluded they were all in bad shape. All were considered diploma mills with understaffing, under-funding and poor quality laboratories and buildings.

The Rockefellers and Carnegies then offered money to correct the situation in those schools that cooperated with them. In return for the money they wanted to be on the board of the schools and determined textbooks, curriculum and other important aspects of the medical programs. The schools that accepted became the prestigious medical schools in the United States and all but one of those who declined the offer disappeared.

As a result of these changes the following was observed: 1) the technical quality of medical education was improved; 2) the curriculum was geared toward drugs and drug therapy; 3) the treatment of choice for most illnesses included drugs; 4) the system was not competitive because drugs are locked in; 5) most physicians knew little about nutrition and natural therapies because it was not included; 6) research continued to be carried out on drugs for cancer therapy. Thus, the triad of surgery, chemotherapy, and radiation remain a strong part of cancer treatment and research and the anti-quackery laws continue to be used against well-meaning physicians. The patient pays a high price for caustic invasive therapy that has a low success rate for survival and those related to the cancer care industry continue to make a lot of money in this multi-billion dollar industry. This money can be seen well beyond the drug companies and physicians to include hospital wings for cancer, continuation of numerous local and national cancer organizations, and even legislators who are rewarded for favors received. If the public were aware of the successful integrative cancer cures available the multibillion-dollar structure would crumble and, thus, the status quo is perpetuated. Another interesting book on the politics involved in cancer written by Daniel Haley (2003) is titled *Politics in Healing: The Suppression and Manipulation of American Medicine.*

In the foreword to *Knockout* (Somers, 2009) Dr. Julian Whitaker uses a different concept for why we are where we are in cancer treatment but reaches the same conclusion. He states, "Conventional medicine's approach to cancer prevention and treatment is a debilitating, often deadly fraud. The physicians who perpetuate this fraud must bear some responsibility, but the problems run much deeper than individual doctors. The underlying issue is that the entire cancer treatment 'industry' has been following a faulty paradigm for close to a hundred years." He further says, "It's clear this approach doesn't work. Over the past hundred years the death rate from cancer has hardly budged, and it will soon be the number one cause of death. Yet, the trillions of dollars vested in its perpetuation have created a powerful and virulent force against change."

In his new book, *White Coat, Black Hat: Adventures on the Dark Side of Medicine* Carl Elliott (2010) says medical trials that were once carried out by medical schools and teaching hospitals have moved to the private sector and drug companies manipulate the research and review boards to get the results they want. After drugs are released they again manipulate the system to get the drugs recognized on the market even if the risk to patients outweighs the benefits. Doctors and their staff are given gifts to encourage the use of the drugs with patients and money is spent to market the drugs directly to consumers. The process is all to make money for the drug companies with little concern for the safety of the consumer. This process has also contributed to the continuation of the triad of cancer care by traditional medicine.

More recently there was research to evaluate overuse of chemotherapy. DeSouza, J. (2011) found that at least one in eight patients in a sample of over 1,000 colon cancer patients where it had metastasized to distant sites received chemotherapy treatments that weren't supported by evidence from clinical trials or by clinical practice guidelines. This was at a significant expense and risk to the patient without proven benefits. The researchers focused on three specific treatments. One had insufficient data to support its use, one had been shown to be ineffective, and one was not supported by data or a compelling rationale. Of the 140 patients receiving unproven chemotherapy there were 869 cycles of chemotherapy with some subjects received two or move unproven treatments. Specifically, 91 of the study patients had 632 intravenous cycles of bevacizumab, at an estimated cost of 1.3 million dollars with potential side effects of hypertension, heightened risk of bleeding and bowel perforation. Fifty-nine subjects received 218 non-evidenced based cycles of capecitabine at an estimated cost of over 600,000 dollars, and potential side effects of diarrhea, nausea, vomiting, fatigue, rash and swelling of the hands and feet. Last, six subjects received 19 cycles of panitumumab at a cost of around 70,000 dollars with potential side effects of itching, dermatitis, and rash. This is a good start at looking at the overuse of chemotherapy.

The Tides are Changing

Changes are coming about in cancer care and more people are using integrative care for a variety of reasons. Some of these reasons follow.

Cost of Traditional Care

First the cost of cancer and all health care continues to increase dramatically and those who have insurance often cannot afford the co-payments and other fees. In addition, it was reported that 86.7 million Americans were uninsured in 2007–2008 (Families, USA, 2009). Statistically at least 15.3% of the population is completely uninsured (US Census, 2008; Families USA, 2009; Americans at Risk, 2009) and a substantial additional portion of the population (35%) is 'underinsured' or not able to cover the costs of their medical needs (Kaiser Commission, 2002, CNN Money, 2009)). Thus, there are economic factors influencing changes in cancer treatment and all health care.

Expanded Groups of Providers and Researchers

A second factor influencing the use of integrative care is the acceptance of and increases in the number of naturopathic physicians, chiropractors, nutritionists and others who are providing cancer information and care outside the area of surgery, chemotherapy and radiation. These therapies are also being researched and reported in professional and lay journals giving them more legitimacy.

National Center for Complementary and Alternative Medicine
A third force leading to change is the National Center for Complementary and Alternative Medicine (NCCAM) established in 1998 as the Federal Government's lead agency for scientific research on the diverse medical and health care systems, practices, and products that are not generally considered part of conventional medicine. This agency provides a degree of legitimacy to alternative treatment and research.

Increased Public Awareness and Use of Integrative Cancer Care

Another force for change is the public who are becoming aware of the poor prognosis of traditional treatment and the opportunities for the less toxic, natural alternative/integrative treatments. The outcome for lung cancer from traditional treatments was presented earlier and is repeated here for emphasis. The relative 5-year survival rates for small cell lung cancer is around 21% if found early and is localized within the lung without any spread to lymph nodes. This category comprises about 6% of all small cell cancer patients. If there are any signs of its spreading to other sites the small cell relative 5-year survival rate is about 11%. This accounts for about 34% of the small cell cancer patients. If there is extensive disease (stage IV) the survival rate is 2%. On the other hand, alternative physicians such as Dr. Forsythe and Dr. Contreras for example, have demonstrated survival rates for stage IV lung cancer that far exceed 2% and may reach upwards to 40 %. And in the past doctors such as Hoxsey claimed an 80% success rate.

Because they are better informed, the public is using more alternative and complementary treatments. For example, in December 2008, the National Center for Complementary and Alternative Medicine (NCCAM) and the National Center for Health Statistics released new findings from the 2007 National Health Interview Survey on Americans use of complementary and alternative medicine (CAM). Information was gathered on 23,393 adults aged 18 years or older and 9,417 children aged 17 years and under. They found that approximately 38% of adults (about 4 in 10) and approximately 12% of children (about 1 in 9) are using some form of CAM in the United States. They were from all backgrounds but CAM use among adults is greater among women and those with higher levels of education and incomes.

Non-vitamin and non-mineral natural products are the most commonly used CAM therapy among adults. The most popular natural products are fish oil/omega 3, glucosamine, Echinacea, and flaxseed. Use has increased for several therapies, including deep breathing exercises, meditation, massage therapy, and yoga but may include acupuncture, ayurveda, biofeedback, chelation therapy, chiropractic or osteopathic manipulations, deep breathing, diet based therapy, energy healing, guided imagery, homeopathic treatments, hypnosis, massage, meditation, movement therapy, natural products such as herbs and products from plants, and enzymes, naturopathy, progressive relaxation, Qi gong, Tai chi, traditional healers such as botanical or native American healers, and yoga.

A recent newspaper article (Associated Press, 2004) listed the ten most common types of alternative medicine used by Americans and the percentage of adults using them. They included: Prayer for own health–43%; Prayer for others–24%; Natural products–19%; Deep breathing exercises–12%; Group prayer–10%; Meditation–8%; Chiropractic care–8%; Yoga–5%; Massage–5%; and Diet-based therapies such as Atkins, Ornish or the Zone–4%. This data was obtained by the Center for Disease Control and Prevention based upon a sample of 31,000 people. The report said over 1/3 of all US adults used some alternative practices in 2002.

Barnes et al (2004) presented results from the National Health Interview Survey on the use of complementary and alternative medicine by the public. This annual survey interviews people nationally about their health and illness-related experiences. The survey included 31,044 adults over age 18 throughout the United States and was designed to be representative of the US population. The study showed that 36% of the population used some sort of complementary and alternative medicine over the past year. When prayers specifically for health reasons were added the percentage of the population using complementary therapies over the past year increased to 62%. In addition, 75% of the sample had used these therapies at some time during their lifetime.

Results similar to those presented above from the National Office of Complementary and Alternative Medicine showed that the five most commonly used therapies are: 1) prayer for self–43%; 2) prayer for others–24.4%; 3) natural products such as herbs and other products from plants and enzymes but excluding vitamins and minerals–18.9%; 4) deep breathing–11.6%; and 5) prayer group–9.6%. These were followed by: 6) meditation–7.6%; 7) chiropractic–7.5%; 8) yoga–5.1%; 9) massage–5%; and 10) diets such as vegetarian, macrobiotic, Atkins, Pritikin, Ornish, or Zone–3.5%. For a further discussion of the results, the reader can review the complete study of 20 pages at www.nccam.nih.gov/news/camsurvey.

Other Factors Influencing the Use of Alternative Therapies for Cancer

Other factors causing the public to consider using alternative complementary therapies are: 1) more pioneering physicians using successful complementary therapies and receiving publicity such as Dr. Francisco Contreras and Dr. James Forsythe who have chapters in this book; 2) more exposure to alternative complementary treatment for cancer by celebrities such as the book *Knockout: Interviews with Doctors Who Are Curing Cancer* by Suzanne Somers; and 3) the computer and social media sites that include groups publicizing alternative treatments. For example, on Facebook, there is a site for cancer that has 953,521 members and several discussion groups with alternative treatments being one of the most active with 75 posts; two groups on vitamin B17 with 1,155 and 1,056 members respectively; and a new lung cancer site with 49 members. The fourth factor is the dissemination of research findings including alternative treatments by computer sites such as MedScape and ScienceDaily Health headlines.

We still have a long way to go in making safe alternative complementary treatments for lung cancer available to the people of the United States. First, the cost of alternative cancer care although usually cheaper than traditional care can still be costly and many insurance plans do not cover it; 2) there is still strong resistance from the medical profession and drug companies; and 3) there are still unqualified people offering advice and services for cancer via the Internet and other media sources without the proper credentials which perpetuates the concept of quackery. But we are slowly moving to the day when successful non-invasive, non-debilitating treatments for lung cancer will be the treatment of choice for all Americans. I look forward to that day when patients and their families will no longer suffer (physically, mentally, spiritually, financially).

Part II

Experience During and After

Lung Cancer of a 38-Year Survivor

Chapter 2

Holistic Alternative Interventions Used

Introduction

It is hard to believe it has been 38-years since I was faced with the diagnoses of lung cancer at the age of 42 and beat all odds for survival after being given 6 months to live. As I look back on my life and talked with my dear friend recently who was so helpful during that period, she asked me, "What was the purpose of that experience in your life." Without hesitation, we both concluded that the experience was given to me so that I might offer encouragement and help to others faced with a diagnosis of lung cancer. Of course, there were other reasons for having this experience such as improving my lifestyle, and moving closer to God that will be discussed in Chapter 3, but the main one was to help others.

If you know about my background you know I am a registered nurse with a doctorate in public health and wellness so I am well grounded in public health, nursing and holistic health. At the time I was diagnosed I had completed my doctorate in public health at Johns Hopkins University and was teaching graduate and undergraduate nursing students and public health students at a local university. Despite my background or maybe because of it, I found the diagnosis of 6 months to live and the prospects of being disabled for that period, as a result of using orthodox treatment, frightening. Thus, I selected alternative holistic treatments to deal with my lung cancer.

My Personal Story of Lung Cancer
Alerted by a Dream

In July 1974 I awoke from a dream telling me to go for a chest x-ray. I have learned to listen to my dreams because they often guided me on health matters, in problem solving, and with finding things. I, thus, tell friends, that God Speaks. I listen. Do You?

Through daily prayer and meditation, being of service to others in my profession of nursing, and using faith, patience and other spiritual attributes in my daily life I have become more aware when God Speaks.

God Speaks With Me
Over the years I have learned how to recognize God's speaking with me. This direction is available to all of us if we listen for God's voice and develop our spiritual attunement that brings us closer to God.

How does God speak with me? Sometimes it is in dreams. For example prior to the diagnosis of lung cancer, a dream told me to get an x-ray. At another time when I had stopped eating meat and poultry, I dreamed that chickens were flying into my face in the hen house. What could be clearer than that I should eat some poultry or other sources of protein? Sometimes God speaks through a friend. For example, the day I was diagnosed borderline diabetic by my primary physician, I stopped to visit the owner of a health food store and discussed the diagnosis with her. She told me about a mineral, GTF chromium, that would stabilize the blood sugar level. I came home and researched it in my nutrition books and, sure enough, it was identified as a way of stabilizing the blood sugar level and this in combination with other holistic interventions eventually resolved the problem. At another time when I continued to have pain after receiving a variety of medical and physical therapy interventions for a back injury I ran into a friend at an antiques show. I told her about the pain and its effect on my walking. She told me about how chiropractic adjustments had helped her resolve the problem. On another day I ran into another friend who not only suggested using a chiropractor to resolve the pain but also gave me the name of one he had used and who had resolved his problem with pain. I went to the chiropractor for a series of treatments and have been free of pain for several years. However, I also carry out a series of anti-aging exercises daily (see Chapter 9) to maintain my freedom from pain (Helvie, 2007). At other times intuitive hunches suggest ways to resolve health issues or to remain healthy. For example, at another time I had an anal fissure and my doctor prescribed nitroglycerine ointment. I knew this was dangerous and I should not use it. I also knew intuitively I should try vitamin E to heal the fissure. Consequently, I used stool softeners, sitz baths, and broke vitamin E capsules and rub the oil on the fissure during the day. In a few weeks it was healed with no side effects.

How do I know it is God speaking and not a negative force in my life? Over the years I have learned to distinguish the feelings I had when planning an intervention that turned out positive. At such times there is no hesitation and I am strong in my conviction with no wavering. It is more of a behavioral response and a feeling of calmness that tells me God has spoken. This communication has served me well because I am currently age 79 and have no known health problems, my lab results for cholesterol, blood sugar and other tests are normal, and I take no prescribed medications. I am one of the 11% of people over age 65 who do not need prescribed medications; and I am one of the few who have overcome lung cancer despite the six months to live sentence of my physician 38 years ago. From remaining healthy most of my life and overcoming conditions such as lung cancer and diabetes by listening to God, I have learned I should listen because the outcome will be positive. These experiences have strengthened my faith and belief in God.

In Chapter 9 some exercises are presented that will help you strengthen your faith, patience and other spiritual attributes and behaviors. These may help you hear God when guidance is offered.

And never underestimate the power of prayer. The following true story will show you how powerful prayer is and should provide a laugh. This was sent to me by email from a friend and there was no information on the author other than the name Dwight Nelson, who recently told a true story about the pastor of his church. He had a kitten that climbed a tree in his backyard and then was afraid to come down. The pastor coaxed, offered warm milk and so forth. The kitty would not come down. The tree was not sturdy enough to climb so the pastor decided that if he tied a rope to his car and pulled it until the tree bent down he could then reach up and get the kitten. That's what he did, all the while checking his progress in the car. He then figured if he went just a little bit further the tree would be bent sufficiently for him to reach the kitten. But as he moved the car a little further forward the rope broke.

The tree went 'boing' and the kitten instantly sailed thorough the air out of sight. The pastor felt terrible. He walked all over the neighborhood asking people if they'd seen a little kitten. Nobody had seen a stray kitten. So he prayed, "Lord, I just commit this kitten to your keeping." And he went on about his business.

A few days later he was at the grocery store and met one of his church members. He happened to look into her shopping cart and was amazed to see cat food. This woman was a cat hater and everyone knew it so he asked her, "Why are you buying cat food when you hate cats so much?"

She replied, "You won't believe this," and then told him how her little girl had been begging her for a cat but she kept refusing. Then a few days before the child had begged again so the mom finally told the little girl, "Well, if God gives you a cat, I'll let you keep it." She told the pastor, "I watched my child go out in the yard, get on her knees and ask God for a cat. And really, Pastor, you won't believe this but I saw it with my own eyes. A little kitten suddenly came flying out of the blue sky with its paws spread and landed right in front of her." So never underestimate the Power of God and His unique sense of humor. He is always there to help when we need it, if we ask.

Medical Attention

When I contacted my physician and asked for a referral for an x-ray he asked if I had symptoms. I told him no, but insisted on a referral and he sent me for x-rays. As a conservative traditional physician, he would not have understood about the guidance offered in dreams and I did not mention this. But I was persistent in my request for an x-ray.

After receiving the x-ray report my physician called and asked me to come to his office. There he told me they found a spot on my lungs that was not there 6 months before and asked that I go into the hospital for a biopsy.

Hospitalization and Diagnosis

Following the lung biopsy while still in the hospital my physician reported that it was a malignant tumor and I needed immediate surgery. He had also arranged for a surgeon to talk with me. I told both physicians I was not willing to rush into any decision about surgery, but wanted all of the information available so I could go home, pray, think about it, and make a rational decision. He told me I would be dead in 6 months without immediate surgery and repeated this several times. I reminded him that the decision about surgery and the responsibility for my life was mine and his responsibility was to give me the information available to help me make a decision.

I believe many patients are so frightened by a diagnosis of cancer and have such faith in their doctor that they do not respond as I did in this situation. Yet, I believe it is your right as a patient to solicit the information and to make your decision based upon what you believe is right for you.

I also believe the doctor in his concern for his patients may give a 3 month or 6 month prognosis to patients to impress upon them the severity of the condition as mine did, but I believe this may be a disservice. For some it may be a self-fulfilling prophecy in which the patient, believing he will die, actually does at the appointed time. I also believe 3 months to live is not a medical diagnosis. I receive many emails from lung cancer patients who have been given such a prognosis. I always respond that 3 months to live or 6 months to live is not a medical diagnosis. It is a GOD diagnosis and only GOD knows when we will die. I then proceed to tell them that I was given that diagnosis 38 years ago and I am still here so it is not always correct. I then offer the person who has emailed me a copy of my ebook that discusses my treatment and recovery, and resources they might consider for treatment whether they choose traditional, complementary or alternative.

Making a Decision

After receiving the diagnosis I consulted a variety of people including family and friends. It is always amazing to me that when you need help making a decision, people appear that fill in all of the pieces. It is like the old adage that when the pupil is ready, the teacher will appear. I call this God speaking with me that was discussed earlier.

My nursing colleagues were traditional medical oriented and wanted the best for me which they saw as surgery. My mother who loved me dearly and was also traditionally oriented said, "Why don't you have surgery and then do the other things." Others did not know what to say so they tried to ignore me at a time when I was most in need of support because of the diagnosis.

Support During the Decision Making

And that support was forthcoming. I spoke with Ursula who was in my Search for God Group. A non-denominational group interested in developing spiritually these groups use material from the Edgar Cayce readings, meet weekly, and study and apply concepts on spiritual attributes such as patience, forgiveness, and love in their daily lives. The group members also select a time to meditate and meditate together daily at each member's home at the selected time. At their weekly meetings members discuss successes and failures in applying the concepts chosen for practice and read material compiled by a group interested in becoming better people who worked over a period of time with Edgar Cayce and who then put the material together in book form. Members of these groups are usually more progressive in thinking and more supportive of others who walk a different path. Thus, I was not surprised that Ursula supported any decision I made and offered her assistance. Through her contacts she was able to obtain a psychic reading from someone in Florida who she believed to be one of the best psychics in the country. His reading was done at a distance so I did not need to travel to Florida. Ursula also agreed to pray about, meditate, and watch her dreams for guidance about the best course of action for my health concern.

Ursula was also available at any time day or night to talk when needed. This was especially important when others tried to put a doubt in my mind about any alternatives other than surgery. Although I rarely needed to talk with Ursula, I valued this offer because I knew that remaining optimistic was very important in recovery from any illness. I also knew the value of support in recovery because support was one of the three components of a healthy resolution of crises situations whether physical or emotional.

Ursula also introduced me to several people locally who had successfully used laetrile (vitamin B17 or amygdaline) as an alternative method of treatment for cancer and gave me the name of a physician in northern Virginia who had successfully treated many patients with it. He was successful at the National Cancer Institute until they were closed because of pressure from the medical and drug organizations. Thereafter, he opened a private practice in northern Virginia and continued to treat with laetrile receiving patients by word of mouth. Like other patients I was required to sign a form that I would not sue or report him.

My plan to forgo surgery and use alternative treatments was based upon: 1) the reading from the psychic who independently identified the tumor and advised against surgery; Instead, he advocated alternative treatments such as laetrile, vitamins, a special diet, stress management, meditation, visualization, and a positive attitude. He said these would resolve the problem. 2) An analysis of Ursula's and my dreams that also concurred and reinforced using an alternative approach. 3) An intuitive knowing that this was the right approach and that God had alerted me and would continue to provide direction and resources for recovery.

Treatment – Physical Aspects

Initially, I contacted the physician in northern Virginia. During my appointment, he examined me, verified the diagnosis of lung cancer, and prescribed a four-prong program. This usual plan included: 1) B-17, amygdaline or the more generic 'nitriloside' or the more popular name 'laetrile', administered by intravenous injections varying from 3 to 9 or more grams, or tablets of 500 mg for oral administration, or available from natural sources such as apricot kernels, millet, fruit and berry seeds, and several beans, seeds, and grains. 2) Nutritional Supplements. 10 or 12 vitamins and minerals administered orally in tablets and capsule form in massive amounts and two or three pancreatic enzyme supplements in the form of panagamic acid. 3) Diet: Mainly fresh uncooked fruit, vegetables, grains and nuts. Avoidance of animal protein, including dairy foods that produce a heavy demand on pancreatic enzymes that are required for effective use of vitamins. 4) Detoxification and maintenance of free and thorough digestive and elimination processes through frequent fasting and or enemas that were considered important for elimination of toxic residue from the breakdown of diseased tissues and for liver stimulation. A minimum program requires an occasional fast for a day or two, ingesting only fruit and vegetable juices, and regular use of supplementary tablets such as comfrey-pepsin and betaine. My specific plan follows.

Amygdaline (Vitamin B17 or laetrile)
My plan included amygdaline (laetrile) 1000 mg in tablet form at bedtime, and one with breakfast and one with lunch (500 mg) for a total of 2000 mg daily. I also carried apricot kernels, the substance from which laetrile is made, and ate about 30 of these periodically during the day as prescribed by the doctor. They are very bitter but I learned to tolerate them by drinking water immediately after. In fact, the water actually tasted sweet after the kernels.

I purchased my amygdaline in Maryland at a pharmacy identified by my physician (neither are in business now) because it was illegal and otherwise unobtainable to my knowledge. However, I did locate some locally when discussing my treatment with a storeowner but it was twice the price I was paying in Maryland. Each month I purchased my amygdaline and paid about $114 a month according to receipts I have saved. Vitamins and enzymes were extra but the total cost was around $200 a month if I remember correctly. I continued amygdaline and the supplements for 2 years. I recently saw prices quoted on the Internet for £490 to £650 for Phase 1 (first 21 days of treatment) and £1,320 to £1,500 for Phase 2 (subsequent 3 months) for amygdaline, vitamins, enzymes and so forth. On another site I recently found 500 mg tablets for $97.50 for 100 that would last for 25 days using the dose I was prescribed.

Periodically after stopping amygdaline I tried to locate apricot kernels for friends who wanted them for cancer but none were available in local stores or later on the Internet. Recently, these have reappeared locally and on the Internet and I recently started taking 10 a day as a preventive measure.

Mechanism of Laetrile. Dr. Ernst T. Krebs, Sr. MD started working to develop laetrile in 1923 and his sons Ernst T. Krebs, Jr. PhD, and Bryon Krebs, MD joined him in his research and perfected it in 1952. A simplified version of the theory advanced by Krebs and discussed by Richardson (1977) is that cancer is a result of malfunctioning of normal mechanisms in the body. Malfunctioning results from a deficiency in a chemical substance found in certain foods and a deficiency in certain enzymes produced in the pancreas. The deficient natural foods are those containing the chemical is nitriloside or vitamin B17 and the deficient pancreatic enzymes are trypsins.

Vitamin B17 contains cyanide but only gives it up in the presence of an enzyme group called beta glucosidase or glucoronidase and this enzyme group is found primarily in cancer cells. When it is found elsewhere in nature it is always accompanied by greater quantities of another enzyme known as rhodanese that converts the cyanide into harmless substances. Cancer cells do not have this protective enzyme and consequently face a double threat, that is the one enzyme when present causes them to be exposed to cyanide, and at the same time the absence of the other enzyme found in other human cells causes a failure to detoxify. Consequently, cancer cells cannot withstand the cyanide in the vitamin B17 and are destroyed because of the composition of their enzymes. On the other hand, normal non-cancer cells are not threatened by the cyanide in vitamin B17 and actually convert it into nutritional substances necessary for health. Because of changes in the production and distribution processes of the current food supply, modern man does not obtain this needed nutrient, vitamin B17, from food, as did earlier generations.

It is believed that the food factor and enzymes were made to work together so the enzymes are equally important. The enzyme trypsinogen is converted to trypsin in the intestines where it is used in combination with chymotrypsin to digest animal protein. Any surplus is absorbed into the bloodstream and digests or dissolves a protein coating that protects cancer cells from the body's defense – the white blood cells. After dissolving this coat the white blood cells are able to move in on the cancer cells and destroy them. However, if the pancreas is weak or exhausted from metabolizing too much sugar, or if the diet contains too much animal protein, then the enzyme is deficient to carry out that process. Thus, Krebs believed cancer was a deficiency disease because it was caused by a deficiency of a vitamin, B17, pancreatic enzymes, or both. The addition of pancreatic enzymes and the altered diet as part of treatment supported this theory.

Other Supplements
The doctor also prescribed a variety of vitamins and minerals, and pancreatic enzymes. **Enzymes** included Wobe Mogus (an enzyme from Germany) 1000 mg 3 tablets at bedtime for one week, then one tablet daily for one week, and then one tablet daily for 6 days a week; Bromelain (ananase) 100 mg 3 tablet before breakfast and dinner, Viokase (pancreatic) and chymo-typsin (digestive) enzymes.

Vitamins included Vitamin A: 50,000u 3 two times a day for one week, then 2 two times a day for one week, then one per day. Vitamin C: 5,000 mg taking one tablet 4 times a day of the time release. Vitamin E: 400 iu taking two at breakfast (protects from vitamin A toxicity). Pantothenic Acid: 100 mg taking one with dinner. Yeast tablets take 10 daily, and pangamic acid (vitamin B15) 50 mg daily and vitamin B5 take 1 daily.

Minerals Calcium, magnesium and zinc.

Herbs included: Comfrey-pepsin – 2 tablets each meal as a digestive aid. (Currently people are warned against using this herb. Contact a reliable source for information.)

Other: I was also prescribed one lecithin capsule at breakfast and at dinner.

Although some people currently use shark cartilage, Barley Green, AHCC (active hexose correlated compound and DMSO (dimethyl sulfoxide) as part of their regime I did not use these. Some think amygdalin has changed in quality over the past 38 years because of the polluted environment including the soil and consequently other supplements may be needed to compensate for these changes.

Diet

The prescribed diet was restrictive with primarily fruit, vegetables and grains. The major things to be omitted were *animal protein* including all meat (beef, pork, fish, poultry), all *dairy products* (milk, cream, cheese), and *simple sugar*. Previously limited amounts of fish and poultry were allowed but experience showed that many seriously ill patients were unable to handle this added metabolic load especially when there was extensive neoplastic involvement. In addition, the physicians who used this regime observed that patients who did consistently well followed the limited diet with no animal protein or sugar. The primary reasons for restricting animal protein are: 1) protein requires the greatest amount of time and chemical energy of all nutrients for digestion and assimilation. In patients with advanced metabolic disease it is preferable to supply the necessary amino acids in tablet form and rely upon other sources such as carbohydrates for energy production. 2) If the digestive system (including liver and pancreas) is not functioning properly, as is often the case in cancer patients, animal protein may be incompletely digested and undergo putrefaction. Thus, some toxic metabolic by products will be formed instead of amino acids. These substances will further strain an already overloaded liver and interfere with vital biochemical processes in normal tissues. Despite the omission of animal protein from the diet, I received an adequate intake of essential amino acids from the fruit and vegetables and from the tablets (Ag/Pro) prescribed by my physician.

Guidelines for the diet included: 1) Use fruits, vegetables, grains – fresh, unprocessed, uncooked. 2) Avoid animal products: because protein diverts pancreatic enzymes needed for processing and assimilation of the vitamins. 3) Uncooked foods should comprise 75% *of the diet* because the critically important enzymes are destroyed at high temperatures.

Use much of the following: fresh fruit-uncooked. Eat two lemons daily. You may also eat apples, pears, grapes, berries, apricots, plums and so forth with seeds and kernels. Citrus fruits can be eaten but no seeds including pineapple. Puree in a blender and keep in the refrigerator or cut up a mixed fruit salad and keep on hand. Also bananas, dates, raisins, prunes, figs, and avocado are good to keep up your weight because they are higher in calories.

Fresh uncooked vegetables can include tomato, carrot, cabbage, cauliflower, beets, turnip, celery, onions, garlic, rutabaga, squash, zucchini, spinach, cress, broccoli, parsley, potato, lettuce, asparagus etc. A juicer is an expensive but important tool for juicing vegetables and combinations can be tried with a basic carrot and celery base. A good basic salad sauce is 2 parts of olive oil and 1 part lemon whipped until creamy.

Vegetables (cooked) can be used but only in addition to ample uncooked vegetables. These may include lima beans, flat beans, legumes, lentils, split peas, artichoke, broccoli, plus any of those listed above under uncooked.

Nuts may include almonds, cashews, walnuts and so forth but *no peanuts* which are a high source of protein. *Grains* and *seeds* may also be used but preferably raw. Several grains can be soaked in water and mixed with other ingredients. Some include millet (rich nitriloside source), buckwheat, oats, brown rice, wheat berries, bulgur, mung beans, barley, alfalfa, sesame, sunflower seeds, pumpkin seeds, wheat germ. Cereals can also be eaten using whole grain and milled non-processed grains without sugar, milk, or salt. Familia Swiss is a good formula. Breads may be used if natural grain, whole grain or sprouted except when white flour, sugar, milk, or salt is included as ingredients. Brewer's yeast (debittered) is good for vegetable protein and several important vitamins and minerals.

Use some of the following foods in this diet. Yogurt can be used on cereal in moderation. Cashew butter can be used in small amounts if natural and without salt or chemicals. Almond milk can be used as a substitute for real milk (forbidden) on cereal. This can be made by adding 8 blanched almonds and 2 tsp of sesame seeds to 8 oz of water and blend thoroughly at a high speed. Chill and use promptly. A limited amount of unsalted butter is permissible. Also a minimal amount of sea salt but no regular salt is allowed. Oils can be used in limited amounts such as olive oil, safflower oil, sesame, unrefined corn oil but no soy oil. Herbal tea was permitted and mayonnaise and carob powder in very limited amounts, Tahini paste was also permissible in limited amounts.

The following foods were *prohibited*: No sugar, or refined sugar products. Animal and animal products, milk, cheese, eggs, and meat were prohibited. However, small portions of fish and poultry may be added after three or four months of the rigorous diet. In addition, occasional eggs or cheese may be permitted at that time. No preservatives, artificial color, or flavors were allowed and that eliminated canned goods. Also, no strong spices, stimulants such as coffee, tea (except herbal tea), alcohol, cigarettes, or chocolate, no tranquilizers, sedatives, or analgesics, and no soy products because of their high protein content.

Amino acid (Ag/Pro) three to nine tablets were allowed daily to compensate for the reduced intake of protein. I took three tablets with meals and I found this necessary because at one point I started to show signs of protein deficiency. After starting the amino acid as well as predigested protein the symptoms resided.

Detoxing

As recommended by my doctor I fasted with fruit and vegetable juices for a day or two each month. I was also on comfrey-pepsin daily so this was already part of my plan of care.

Exercise

Although my doctor did not discuss exercise I knew it was important for maintaining weight and other aspects of health so I continued daily walking on the beach at the Atlantic Ocean. This not only allowed me exercise but also provided diversion by watching the tourists in the busy resort area where I lived. Current research demonstrates the value of exercise in many types of cancer prevention and treatment so perhaps God was nudging me in my program of care. It might be of interest to also say that despite the restricted diet I did not lose weight and at some point actually had to limit my intake of fruit to avoid excessive gaining.

Smoking Cessation

As a cigarette smoker and knowing that this accounts for most of the lung cancer cases, it was necessary to do something about this unhealthy behavior. I initially reduced smoking to fewer cigarettes with less tar and nicotine but knew I had to quit. This is a difficult process but I accomplished it following some of the techniques identified in Chapter 9 and outlined on my CD on smoking cessation.

Mental and Spiritual Aspects of Treatment

Although my doctor was vague about other aspects of treatment, I had worked with alternative treatments for years, had read extensively on such methods as meditation, visualization, and the influence of prayer, and had worked several years with the Edgar Cayce methods as a volunteer camp nurse at the Cayce Camp during my summer vacations from teaching nursing. Thus, I developed the following regime to supplement the prescribed physical interventions. The interested reader is referred to Chapter 10 for a more detailed discussion on the specific steps in how to carry out these interventions and the research related to them.

Visualization

Visualization was an important part of my regime. Each day I spent two fifteen-minute sessions in a quiet setting with my eyes closed and visualized the cancer cells being reduced by the laetrile and vitamins and disappearing from my body by being carried out of my body with other waste products. At other times I imagined fresh healthy air with energy entering my body as I inhaled and cancer cells leaving as I exhaled. I also visualized my body as healthy and congratulated myself for being successful. I continued this for two years and periodically thereafter, if needed.

Meditation

I also meditated for 30 minutes each evening before I retired. At the start of each meditation I focused on a positive affirmation such as "Lo I am with You Always, Even Till the End" and then emptied my mind of all thoughts. When thoughts intruded I again returned to the affirmation and the emptying process. Because I had spent many years in the Search For God group based upon the Edgar Cayce work with those interested in becoming better people, I used the Cayce approach to meditation. In the books that are used by these groups there are affirmations for each chapter that follow the spiritual attributes and concepts being used such as patience, forgiveness and brotherly love. Some of the affirmations closely follow biblical passages and those work well also. Whatever I used was used to focus my mind to allow God to speak to me and also to help me remain positive. The reader will remember my discussion earlier of God speaking with us when we are attuned to him. I also continued my weekly Search for God meetings and meditated daily with this group.

Affirmations and Stress Management

During the day I also used positive affirmations as often as possible. A typical affirmation might be "I am happy and healthy and God is with me". At stressful times I practiced stress management techniques. For example, if there was stress in situations encountered during my daily teaching I retreated to my office and, after quieting my body, visualized a peaceful setting, meditated briefly, or went through progressive relaxation exercises. The reader will recognize that stress management is a combination of mental/spiritual processes. All will be discussed in Chapter 10.

Maintaining a Positive Attitude

One of the most important aspects of my regime was to maintain a positive attitude toward daily life and recovery. If others talked about following the doctor's orders for surgery or in any way placed a doubt in my mind, I thanked them for their concern and walked away. If necessary, my friend Ursula was always available to talk, give support, and renew my confidence in my approach. At such times I might also meditate, pray, use an affirmation or visualize something positive.

I learned a positive attitude from my mother who had cancer when I was in high school. Her cancer was in the cervix of the uterus and she was treated with radium and x-ray. When she recovered and returned home her family doctor told her he did not think she would live to get to the hospital. She said she knew the family did not expect here to live but was surprised about her doctor. She also said she had to live because she had three children in school and had to get home and see them graduate. With that attitude she lived many more years.

I believe another important aspect of being optimistic and positive is a result of spiritual activities in my life. It is easier to be optimistic of a positive outcome of cancer or any illness if you have faith in a higher being to guide you through rough times.

Prayer

In addition to my own daily prayers, I contacted several friends who added me to prayer lists in their churches. I also contacted the Glad Helpers at the Association for Research and Enlightenment and was added to their daily prayer list. In addition, I contacted the now deceased Olga Worrall, a nationally known psychic healer, who put me on her healing list and prayed for me each day. I had read about Olga and her husband Ambrose for years and was reassured after talking with her. And when I called her, it was like she was expecting my call and that was nice.

For those unfamiliar with Olga and Ambrose Worrall, they were psychic from early childhood, met, fell in love and devoted their life to helping others. Living in Baltimore, Maryland, they were founders of the New Life Clinic that continues to operate today and can be reached at PO Box 65070, Baltimore, Maryland 21209. A form for requesting prayers can be found at http://www.thenewlifeclinic.com/joinprayerlist.php. An interesting story of their life and work can also be found in *The Gift of Healing* (Worrall, 1977).

I am not religious but consider myself a very spiritual person with a strong faith and belief in a higher being that for me is Jesus and God having been raised in a Christian home. However, I believe in the power of prayers to Buddha, Allah and other spiritual beings and also believe this is an important part of any cancer treatment.

Other Spiritual Interventions

I continued working daily as a nurse educator during my treatment and tried to be of service to others and I consider this an important spiritual quality. I also strengthened my faith, patience, forgiveness and other spiritual characteristics that I consider important in one's life and healing process.

Other Holistic Treatments

As a nurse with a public health background I practiced a holistic approach to care of clients so I applied this concept in my own life. In addition to the physical, mental and spiritual concepts discussed above I also believed the environment, relationships, and politics are important because these all influence health and in this instance cancer. A summary of the total treatment program I followed will give an idea of some of these holistic activities.

Physical Aspects: diet; exercise; vitamins; laetrile; apricot pits, smoking cessation.

Mental Aspects: meditation; visualization; relaxation; remaining positive; replacing negative thoughts with positive ones.

Spiritual Aspects: faith in a higher being; strengthening my patience, faith and forgiveness; being of service to others; emotional support from a friend; church prayerlists: psychic healer, prayers.

Environmental: smoke-free environment; no pesticides, no mold or other chemicals; aired my house when possible; emergency medical numbers posted.

Relationships: maintained friendships with students, colleagues, friends, and family and received support (increases probability of recovery) from them.

Politics: active in publishing, and lecturing, about complementary approaches to cancer; active in professional organizations to help bring about change in health care (inclusion of complementary alternative practices and health care for all people).

Outcome of Cancer Treatment

Although the cancer specialist did not ask me to return I visited my primary physician every three months. I did not tell him about my therapy because I knew he would not understand or accept it. He thought I was in a wait and see mode. However, I visited him for x-rays to determine if there were any changes in the size or location of the tumor. I did not allow him to discuss surgery and reminded him, if necessary, that I was responsible for my life.

I continued my treatment and visits to my physician for two years after which time the tumor was gone. My local physician said he thought he must have made an incorrect diagnosis but a physician friend who was the head of Blue Cross and Blue Shield in another state and who I had previously taught with in a well-known southern university reviewed all of the lab reports, biopsy, x-rays, and other tests and concluded that it had definitely been lung cancer based upon the biopsy and x-ray reports. He also concurred that the tumor was gone.

Comments for Those with Symptoms or Newly Diagnosed

I would like to end this chapter with some comments to those who may have symptoms or are faced with a diagnosis of lung cancer. If you have symptoms of lung cancer please see your physician immediately to obtain a diagnosis. This could save your life.

If you are diagnosed and considering conventional treatment consult your doctor and ask him/her about a treatment plan, the pros and cons of conventional treatment, what you can expect from treatment, what are the side effects and does he have ways to deal with these or utilize a naturopathic physician to deal with the side effects, what is your prognoses and other questions you may have. If you are considering using alternative treatment seek out Dr. Contreras, Dr. Forsythe or one of the other competent physicians who are successfully treating lung cancer and ask them similar questions. Consult family and friends. Then YOU make the decision using all of the information you obtained because the decision is yours to make. Consult an alternative physician about alternative treatments. Don't underestimate the power of prayers; pray for guidance. This could lead to dreams or intuition that might help you make a decision about what is best for you. Once you make a decision about the treatment, you need to stay positive about your treatment and the choices you have made. Research shows a definite relationship between being positive and health outcomes. And consider a holistic approach to care that involves the six areas I used which include physical, mental, spiritual health, the environment, relationships, and politics. Although politics are important this is an area of holistic health that can be delayed when dealing with a new diagnosis of lung cancer.

As a lung cancer survivor who has a strong faith in God, and as a nurse I like to help others when possible so remember I am also here to help. Do not hesitate to contact me with any questions or comments you may have. I will be happy to share information and resources and to add you to my prayer list, if desired. Over the years of dealing with my own personal cancer experience including preventing a recurrence and responding to others who need help, I have learned about and interacted with many of the brave successful physicians who have bucked the system to do what is right and to increase the potential of survival for patients. I am always happy to share these resources with you.

Chapter 3

Holistic Interventions to
Prevent Recurrence

Introduction

It has been 36 years since my lungs were clear from cancer and I have been free of any signs of a recurrence. Research indicates that a healthy lifestyle is important to prevent a recurrence of cancer and I have tried to live one in my daily life. Using a wellness focused holistic approach to life I have not only remained free of cancer but also remained very healthy. For example, at age 79 I have no chronic illnesses and no prescribed medications. The average for a 75 year old is three chronic illnesses and 5 prescribed medications and, in addition, current statistics show that only 11% of all people over age 65 in the United States are free of chronic illnesses and prescribed medications. So I am one of the minorities of the population in that group and it has been because of my lifestyle, I believe.

I am very active physically living in a 3-story house where I am up and down stairs during the day, and walk at least 3 miles on the beach at 7:00 in the morning. I am also active mentally locating and interviewing guests, editing each program, and hosting a radio show on Holistic Health. I also write articles, a monthly newsletter and work on my current book that takes several hours each day. I also find time for God each day with prayers and meditation and for my fellow man with quick responses to questions about cancer or other health concerns. I believe all of these activities are extremely important.

In this chapter I will remember as best I can what I have done over the past 36 years that allowed me to remain cancer free since recovering from lung cancer. I continued to use a holistic approach to prevention in my life and will break down my behaviors into the categories used earlier. These are physical, mental, spiritual, relationships, environmental, and politics.

Physical Aspects
Nutrition and Water

My regime to remain healthy and prevent a recurrence starts with a healthy diet. The diet I chose was less restrictive than the diet used during treatment but followed a similar pattern of many fruits and vegetables and as much raw as possible. However, I added some protein and carbohydrates initially. This has changed over time and all simple sugar has been eliminated for the past several years. Although pie, cake, candy and ice cream are delicious, they are also known from research to feed cancer cells

Fruit and Vegetables

I continued to eat mostly organically grown or local small farmer fruits and vegetables to avoid genetically engineered foods, pesticides, growth hormones and other contaminants. I also try to eat *fresh* fruit and vegetables and avoid canned or frozen or processed foods where preservatives or other additives are added. You can imagine that if food will last for months or years in a can what the can must be coated with to allow this. I prefer not to subject myself to that. I also avoid fresh fruits and vegetables from Mexico and other southern countries. This has made eating fresh during the winter months more difficult so I now freeze organic fruits and vegetables for the winter and eat fresh during the spring and summer months. It sometimes means navigating between Trader Joe's, Fresh Market, the farmers' market, and Harris Teeter's to obtain what I need for this diet. On my cancer diet discussed in Chapter 2, 75% of my fruits and vegetables were raw. Currently with the exception of salads for lunch during the summer months most of my vegetables are cooked.

Protein

I have added some protein to my diet in the form of chicken, occasional fish and seafood, cheese, and small amounts of milk. I have not eaten beef for over 20 years and never eat farm-grown salmon because of toxins, but I do eat wild caught salmon. I limit my fish and seafood to one or two times a week because of mercury and other pollutants. I eat chicken and cheese most days. Milk is used on cereal at breakfast but rarely used otherwise. Eggs are eaten occasionally and pork is rarely eaten.

Grain and Nuts

I eat cereal for breakfast on most days that usually consists of shredded wheat or oatmeal. I rarely eat bread, pasta, potatoes or other starchy foods. I eat many nuts starting with dry roasted pecans on my cereal at breakfast. If I want something after meals in place of fruit I eat some walnuts (good for increasing good cholesterol), cashews, pistachios, macadamia, or almonds.

Simple Carbohydrates

Sugar in the form of cakes, pies, candy and other sweets were my downfall but a few years ago my body and research on sugar and cancer told me it was time to quit so I never eat any of these now. Perhaps once or twice a year I will celebrate with something sweet made without sugar on a special occasion like my birthday or Christmas but that is rare.

Typical Daily Meal Plan

Most breakfasts consist of oatmeal with organic berries (blackberry, raspberry, blueberry, or strawberry) and roasted, salted pecans and a little organic fat-free milk (note that milk is limited and was prohibited during my lung cancer treatment discussed in Chapter 2). About six months ago I added 12 prunes to breakfast as a stool softener. Almost every lunch consists of a vegetable salad (organic vegetables) with some cheese or chicken (organic) and sugar-free dressing during the summer months. Many days I also have a vegetable soup such as gazpacho. If I eat chicken on my salad I usually eat nuts or cheese at night. Lunch is usually followed with an orange, apple, watermelon or other organic fruit. During the winter months I usually eat vegetable soup made with a variety of organic low and high carbohydrate vegetables. My dinners consist of either cheese, chicken or seafood plus three cooked vegetables such as broccoli, squash and cauliflower, and a piece of fruit. Except for my winter soup I eat primarily low carbohydrate vegetables and avoid the high carbohydrate ones such as potatoes, carrots, and corn. If I am still hungry following the evening meal I eat a handful of nuts or a piece of fruit.

Organic Food
As mentioned earlier I eat as much organic food as I can find. Recently I read an article about the current business of growing chickens. In the article they described how baby chickens are purchased and put in crowded pens where the manure and other excrements are left and the chickens must wade in it. They are given antibiotics to prevent infections and this is pasted on to customers who eat them. It is believed that this accounts for some of the drug resistance we experience. Poultry and other marketable animals may also be given growth hormones to make larger chickens and these may be found in the food as well. Thus, free-range organic chicken becomes a necessity for me to remain free of cancer. In addition, pesticides are often used on fruit and vegetables and/or they may be genetically modified. This makes the food different that it was years ago when I was a child and we grew our own foods before greed entered the marketplace to put a buck before the health of the public. Research on genetically modified foods continues to produce results showing that these foods are not healthy. In addition, the government does not require labeling of genetically modified food so the consumer is

unaware of which are generically modified and which are not. However, organic foods eliminate most of these concerns for me.

It is of interest that many of the complementary physicians providing successful alternative cancer care recommend organic food as part of their plan of care. This reinforces the fact that all of these pollutants, in food which is not organic, are not healthy and should be avoided. Thus, I continue my organic foods and periodically do a short-term detoxification to eliminate any toxins present.

Sugar Substitute
I do not use sugar because of its close relationship to cancer activity, yeast infections, arthritis, obesity, and other health concerns. However, there are times when I want something sweet such as on my cereal. Until a few years ago I used Sweet'N Low that I knew was a carcinogen but I did not know about other sugar substitutes, except NutraSweet which I could not tolerate and which has since been shown from research to be one of the worst chemicals on the market. When I interviewed Dr. Patrick Quillin, a nutritionist, for my radio show he said Stevia was the only sugar substitute one should use because it is an herb. At that time, I began using Stevia and have been very happy to have a substitute that tastes good and that I know is not carcinogenic.

Microwaves, Fast Foods, Barbecues, and TV Dinners
There has been research in the past about the harmful effects of using microwaves for food preparation and I have read that they are banned in Russia because they reduce the nutritional value of food and promote illness. One study showed pathological changes of subjects using microwaves in food preparation including an increase in leukocytes and a decrease in lymphocytes. The study also showed an increase in total cholesterol and a decrease in blood iron levels. In another study of cow's milk exposed to microwaves, there was an increase in acidity, a

change in the structure of the fat molecule, a reduction in folic acid, and an increase in non-protein nitrogen. In a recent experiment carried out by a high school student spring water was heated in the microwave, cooled and put on a jalapeno plant and another pan of water was heated on the stove and cooled and put on another jalapeno plant for four weeks. The plants were kept side-by-side outdoors in the sun and watered equal amounts daily. Signs of growth were also observed daily. At the end of four weeks the plant watered with the water from the microwave had not grown whereas the one from the stovetop water grew rapidly and had a couple jalapenos on it. Afterwards both plants were transplanted into the same larger pot and fed unheated spring water. The plant previously fed stovetop water continued to grow rapidly and produce many jalapenos whereas the plant previously given microwave heated water lost its leaves and died within three days (De Wet, 2010, p 235). As a result of this information, I have put my microwave away and use it only occasionally. I now cook my vegetables in an electric wok and cook oatmeal on top of the stove. It does not take much longer than it did with the microwave.

I have not eaten fast foods for years because of the high fat and sugar content and lack of nutritional value. If I am traveling and there is no other resource available I will stop at a fast food restaurant and order a salad with a salad dressing free of sugar and a low fat content.

Likewise, I never eat food prepared on a grill unless I am at someone's home at mealtime and they serve it. When high fat meat or pork (which I almost never eat) are grilled burning fat drips into the open flames and forms polycyclic aromatic hydrocarbons (PAHs) that contain a variety of carcinogens. Blackened toast and other charred foods are also carcinogens and on the rare instance I might eat toast I scrape any blackening off. I also avoid barbecued foods because of the high fat and sugar content.

TV dinners are also avoided because of the low nutritional

value, the plastic container they are sold in and the need for using the microwave to finish preparing. Heating the plastic may cause it to melt into the food and produces toxin chemicals in the body.

Oils and Salt

I also choose the oils I use in cooking with care to avoid oils that may turn carcinogenic when heated above a certain temperature. Although there is disagreement in the literature, I find that organic extra virgin olive oil has the best report and can be heated to 485 degrees before turning carcinogenic so I use this for cooking. I also use it primarily for salad dressings.

Recently I discovered that table salt also contains chemicals so I have switched to Himalayan crystal salt with ionic minerals. An excellent book that discusses salt and many other lifestyle factors which affect health is *Survive! A Family Guide to Thriving in a Toxic World* (Wynters and Goldberg, 2010). This book is a must for anyone who wants to make changes that will improve his/her health.

The reader might think my food choices are boring or take a lot of time to implement. However, I enjoy the foods on my diet and the resulting improvement in health that allows me to enjoy life without pain, medications, or limitations in physical or mental activities. In addition, I love to be constantly learning new things and I read extensively in the area of health for my radio show and Internet blog on which I post three times a week. I also learn from my guests on my radio show and implement new ideas I learn from them.

Food shopping which I do one day a week may take a little longer but I have met many interesting people and have my weekly visit with clerks and others in the stores I frequent. Food preparation may also take a bit longer than when I used the microwave or ate some fast foods but it tastes so much better. After you eliminate some of the processed foods, sugars, and other harmful aspects of nutrition, your taste buds change and the more nutritious foods taste great.

Water

The scientific literature is controversial about the best water to drink. For years I used distilled water where water is boiled and steam is collected in a condensing unit for drinking. This process removed most of the bacteria, viruses, chemicals, minerals and pollutants. Thus, the water is one of the purest and most satisfactory for drinking. Because this method removed minerals and vitamins, I replaced them with supplements. Water is very necessary to remove toxins from the body and I always drink at least 8 glasses and usually more each day. About a year ago I started drinking two glasses of water as soon as I get up in the morning to replenish that lost during the night. Many older people do not get adequate water and develop dizziness and other symptoms due to dehydration.

A few years ago I read that distilled water also tends to make the body more acidic. That has been one challenge for me because I tend to remain acidic despite my diet and consequently take mineral supplements and lemon to correct this (see the discussion below). As a result of this new information I subsequently reverted to drinking spring water for 6 months and distilled water for two months. Spring water varies in quality and the amount of contaminants removed so I check the labels carefully before using it. Water in plastic containers is also problematic because of the bleeding of the chemicals in the containers into the water when heated during transport in the summer months.

Vitamins, Mineral, and Other Supplements

Vitamins, Minerals, Herbs

I take a variety of vitamins, minerals and other supplements daily. At breakfast I take a multivitamin, one 500 mg bilberry capsule, and two 300 mg calcium tablets. According to the directions three of the multivitamins I take supply all of the daily requirements for iodine for the thyroid and if I drop the dose my thyroid drops below recommended levels. However, the three multivitamins daily maintain the thyroid levels. I started bilberry over 2 years ago when my eye doctor said I had bad cataracts and would need surgery within 6 months. When I returned to his office in 6 months my vision had improved so much that he said surgery was not indicated. I take three of these each day having one with each meal. Within the last year I added one Super Zeaxanthin daily. It contains lutein and is one of the best herbal preparations for eye health. Since taking the bilberry and Super Zeaxanthin my vision has continued to improve, the cataracts are improving, and the floaters in my eyes have disappeared so I am seeing brilliant blues, greens and other colors I had not seen for years. In addition, I do a series of Indian pressure point exercises daily for the eyes.

About three years ago my PSA rose to 9.6 and I started pomegranate elixir. Within two months my PSA was 4.8 and in another month it was 4.0. I take one of these an hour after breakfast each day. Research shows that pomegranate will prevent prostate cancer and if there is a tumor will reduce its size. At the same time I started getting up hourly during the night and my urologist diagnosed BPH (benign prostatic hypertrophy), an enlarged prostate that frequently happens to men at a much younger age. Research shows that fruit and vegetables may delay the onset of BPH and as mentioned earlier I eat a lot of fruit and vegetables. After discussing treatment with my urologist I proposed using natural products for this and he was agreeable. Initially I used beta systosterol that controlled the symptoms for 6 to 8 months. I later switched from this to three pumpkin seed extract capsules, one cranberry extract capsule, one stinging nettle capsule, and three natural prostate capsules containing saw palmetto, pygeum, 5-loxin, lycopene and other herbs each day. About a year ago I began getting up during the night and subsequently added 6 colostrums capsules daily to my BPH regime. Not only did these control the symptoms but they also eliminated my seasonal allergies developed in 2003 after Hurricane Isabel. I should add that these herbs not only control the symptoms very well but I do not need to worry about side effects.

I take most of my daily vitamins and minerals at the lunch meal. These include the second multivitamin, one of the bilberry mentioned earlier, calcium 300 mg, vitamin D 1200 mg, magnesium 300 mg, vitamin E 500 iu, vitamin C 2500 mg, omega 3/6/9/ (borage, fish and flax oils) and an additional flax oil 1000 mg.

At the evening meal I take my last bilberry, one 500 mg quercetin, one seleno-6 100 mcg, and one curcumin 400 mg. All have been shown to have a positive effect on cancer prevention. I also take my final multivitamin then.

Probiotics

About four years ago I developed a severe yeast infection as a result of two series of antibiotics prescribed by my primary physician for what he thought was a prostate infection. At that time I did not know the value of probiotics while on antibiotics nor did my physician. After using a natural treatment for the yeast and recovering I continue with a preventive maintenance program to maintain a healthy intestinal flora. For this I use one packet of three lax or five lax (a probiotic) before breakfast, 7 drops of oxygen element max in a glass of water three times a day, and one capsule of 8 billion acidophilus and bifidus, one capsule of yeast defense, and one flora five, an enteric-coated probiotic, in the afternoon.

Apricot Kernels

For many years I did not take apricot kernels because the FDA removed them from the market as dangerous. Textbooks still perpetuate the myth that they are dangerous and can cause severe damage to the body. Recently they became available on the Internet and locally and I have started 10 a day as a preventive. After taking these for a month I realized I felt much better and had more energy.

Minerals and Nutrition for Alkalinity

About 5 years ago I checked my acid-alkaline base and found I was very acidic despite a diet heavy with fruits and vegetables. At that time I started checking my urine for its acidity more regularly and taking minerals and lemon juice in water to become more alkaline. It is know that cancer cells and yeast overgrowth thrive in an acidic body. It is also known that an acidic body may be a factor in other diseases. For example, Edgar Cayce many years ago said that maintaining an alkaline body would prevent all colds and other conditions.

Cayce said the body should be slightly alkaline. This is obtained from fruits, vegetables, and milk products. Acid producing foods include meats, grains, and sweets. He said everyone should eat an 80% alkaline to 20% acid diet. Beverages in the alkaline diet included milk and milk drinks, ovaltine, herbal teas, vegetable juices, and pure or boiled water (6 to 8 glasses daily).

Foods that should be eaten in moderation included coffee, desserts, fruit, gelatin desserts, ice cream, salt (use kelp, sea or vegetable), and tea with milk or cream.

He said you should avoid certain foods such as animal fat, raw apples, beer, candy, carbonated beverages, condiments, fried foods, hard liquor, pork (except crisp bacon occasionally), white flour, raw or rare meat. You should also avoid certain food combinations such as citrus and cereal or other starches, citrus and milk, coffee or tea with milk, fruit and vegetables at same meal, meat or cheese with starch, raw apple with other food, sweets (sugar) and starch, vegetables cooked with meat or meat fat. I use these concepts in my meal planning. It is interesting that the anti-inflammatory diet prescribed by Dr. Andrew Weil is similar to the Cayce Acid-Alkalinity diet.

Acid-Alkalinity in Cancer Treatment.
It is also interesting that the acid-alkalinity concept is used in cancer treatment. For example, Dr. Nicolas Gonzales (Somers, 2009) bases his current successful treatment for cancer on two types of individuals. These are sympathetic and parasympathetic and the type is related to whether one is acidic or alkaline and will also determine what type of cancer one will develop if these are out of balance. These types will also determine part of one's individualized treatment plan.

According to Dr. Gonzales those who develop lung cancer, for example, are sympathetic and have an acidic body balance. This may explain why I have so much difficulty bringing my body into balance and must use minerals, lemonade and other means to do so.

Medical History over the Years
Despite our efforts to remain healthy we will have health concerns as we age. However, my goal has been to prevent as many health crises as possible and to treat those that occur with as many natural non-invasive procedures as possible in an effort to maintain my immune system and prevent a recurrence of cancer. When necessary I do utilize traditional medicine such as surgery when I had a strangulated inguinal hernia. I also rely heavily on guidance from God on interventions through my dreams, intuition or other means as discussed in Chapter 2. I will now present my medical history and interventions used as best as I can remember.

Over twenty years ago I developed a hernia and discussed this with my physician who failed to identify it. Believing he must be right I participated in an antique show 100 miles from home. It became strangulated and I drove home and to the emergency unit. Thereafter, it was repaired by surgery and has not been problematic since. I used Edgar Cayce's Scar Massage on the incision scar that disappeared and has not been visible for years.

I also had a series of elevated blood sugars about 20 years ago and was diagnosed borderline diabetes. My friend and owner of the health food store told me about glucose factor chromium (a mineral) and I researched it in my nutrition books and found that it did, in fact, stabilize the blood sugar level. I started using 400 mg daily and within two years my three month blood sugar levels were normal and I have not had any further problem. I know that my lifestyle pattern of eating no simple sugars currently and daily exercise also facilitates a normal blood sugar level.

About 15 years ago I arrived at the university where I taught and had one of the nurse practitioner faculty members ask if I felt well. I said yes, why? She said my mouth was drooping. She tested my hand strength and asked a series of questions and told me I had not had a stroke but did have Bell's palsy. She said I should see my primary physician, which I did. He prescribed steroids. However, on my way home I saw another faculty member who told me she had just been to a seminar on Bell's palsy and told me I should try a homeopathic remedy, which I picked up at the local health food store. It was aconitum napellus and causticum. I used these for 10 days and all symptoms were gone. I never filled the steroid prescription.

About 10 years ago I developed severe pain in my abdomen that my primary physician diagnosed as diverticulitis. I was given a prescription for steroids and told to avoid berries, nuts and other foods that could catch in the intestinal pockets. I was also told that I must avoid these foods the rest of my life. On my way home from this appointment I stopped at the health food store and bought a gallon of aloe vera juice. I drank 4 ounces twice a day and within two days the pain was gone. Within a couple weeks I was again eating berries and nuts and have continued to this day with no side effects. In fact, I eat berries daily for breakfast and about 4 pounds of nuts weekly.

When I become lax with my acid-alkalize balance supplements (minerals and lemon) I experience some arthritic pain in my hands and this is resolved by becoming diligent with my program again. However, I am sure that my daily walking, diet, prayer, meditation and other holistic interventions are also important in maintaining my healthy state.

About 8 years ago I was lifting a heavy object and injured my back. I was in so much pain that I did use the prescribed steroids followed by physical therapy recommended by my physician. When physical therapy was completed I still had pain and my physical therapist said it was arthritis and I would have it the rest of my life. I told her I did not have it before the accident and I did not expect to have it permanently now. A friend suggested I try his chiropractor and within one year I was pain free. I have remained this way as long as I do my anti-aging exercises at least 6 days a week. I also learned to locate muscle spasms and release the pain using an Omni massage Roller.

About the same time I developed an anal fissure and my doctor prescribed nitroglycerine ointment. Because this is so dangerous to the body I chose not to use it and was intuitively directed to use vitamin E. Several times daily I squirted the oil from a vegetarian vitamin E capsule and put it on the anal fissure. I also used daily stool softeners and drank 8 ounces of aloe vera daily. Within three months the area was completely healed. I have since started eating 12 prunes with breakfast in place of the stool softeners.

During Hurricane Isabel in 2003 I had three feet of water pass through my house. Although my living space is on the second and third floor of my house, I had many things stored on the first floor and they were destroyed. Without electricity and air conditioning for 10 days everything got moldy and had to be thrown out. In addition, the wallboard had to be removed and replaced up to several feet above the ground. Following this experience I was in a run-down condition and developed severe pneumonia. I was treated with antibiotics and other traditional medicine over a long period and spent a lot of time in bed. Eventually the condition was resolved and I started taking Host Defense 2 capsules daily during the winter months to build my immune system and prevent a recurrence. Host Defense is made from 17 types of organic mushrooms. During the past winter season taking colostrums has eliminated the need for Host Defense.

Shortly thereafter I developed seasonal allergies and was tested and found to be allergic to cats, dogs, dust, feathers, ragweed and other allergies. Because I did not want to take the drugs the doctor prescribed I searched my materials from the Edgar Cayce readings and was reminded of ragweed tincture. I started taking 1 teaspoon once a day and eventually twice a day and all symptoms subsided. At the beginning of the allergy season my left eye would be inflamed when I got up in the morning and I knew it was time to start the ragweed. Within three days the inflammation cleared and I continued to take it twice a day during the allergy season and there were no further symptoms. A couple years ago I increased the ragweed tincture to two teaspoons twice a day. Interestingly, it is effective against most of my allergens but I do not put myself in long-term situations where it would be tested. I usually continue the treatment for two or two and a half months and stop. Until a year ago the irritation occurred spring and fall, but then it was only in the spring. This year there was no allergic reaction in the spring either. I know there are certain foods that reduce allergies, and also building the immune system is important to reduce or prevent the symptoms. Thus, I believe my diet, exercise and other aspects of a holistic lifestyle are important in reducing or eliminating the stimulus that set off the allergies. In addition, the colostrum I take for BPH is an immune builder and probably had a role in the elimination of seasonal allergies this past year.

Once or twice a year I detox my body with essiac tea from Canada. I follow the directions on the bottle for one month each time. Although I try to remain free of chemicals in food and air and avoid medications as much as possible this is not completely possible in our highly polluted environment. Therefore, detoxing is an important part of remaining healthy and preventing a recurrence of cancer. During my cancer treatment I used monthly fasting with only fruit and vegetable juices. Since recovery I did nothing for many years and about 4 years ago started using the essiac tea. This flushes out all of the toxins accumulated in the body from food, air, and water.

Exercise

I have maintained an exercise regime consistently since recovery from lung cancer. Exercises consist of a daily set of anti-aging or Tibetan exercises, walking, weight lifting, and isotonic exercises. The anti-aging exercises are presented in Chapter 10. Weight lifting involves lifting a 2-pound weight in each hand over my head and returning to my side 45 times each morning. Walking ranges from three miles to occasionally 10 miles a day. For the past 10 years I have walked the beach on the Chesapeake Bay for at least three miles most mornings between 6:30 and 7 am except during my recovery from a back injury. The isometric exercises are to maintain my upper body. In addition, for the past 10 years I have lived in a 3-story house so I am up and down stairs often.

Staying Busy

My career has always kept me so busy that I had little time to think about a recurrence of cancer and I believe this has been important in my continuing good health. I was not only busy but I was busy doing things I liked to do and also busy helping others. Initially I was teaching students how to help their patients stay healthy in homes, clinics and community settings. I was also working with a homeless population and involved my students in providing health care for them. Sometimes this involved helping students accept a homeless group who were different from their previous contacts. Sometimes it was helping them problem solve how best to help individuals with their health needs who do not have a permanent home. At one point I received a grant from the Division of Nursing for almost one million dollars to provide primary care for the homeless and low-income populations; established a nursing center; and both administered this program and taught some of the students rotating through the nursing center. I believe helping others was a way of giving back to the world for my life that God saved for a purpose.

I was also busy writing books for students, carrying out research and giving papers around the United States and Europe, assuming leadership positions in local, state and national organizations in nursing and public health and reading research information in order to keep up to date and have information to share with students, patients and colleagues. This not only assisted in keeping me busy but allowed me the opportunity to share with others and advocate for those who were less fortunate than me.

After retiring at the age of 69, I continued my leadership activities with national professional organizations such as the American Public Health Association and Sigma Theta Tau, the nursing honor society, continued research and presenting papers, reading, assisting and advocating for others. In 2007, I published my 7th book and was interviewed on many radio shows. I also began hosting my own radio show where I could reach many people through the education programs presented and through the emails and telephone calls to those who asked for assistance with resources for treatment of cancer. The Internet is a marvelous creation for bring us together and as a result of my radio show, appearing on other shows, and my website those seeking help with cancer often found my site. So with this brief overview of my busy time as I live a holistic lifestyle I hope you can see why this kept me occupied and was helpful in my maintaining my health.

Mental Aspects

Before one picks up a gun and shoots another person (physical act), he must have negative feelings (mental process). Underlying those feelings is his spiritual foundation that allows him to harbor those negative thoughts or avoid them. Because our health results from interrelated physical, mental and spiritual interactions it is necessary to work with all of these in order to improve health and life. It is well-known that you cannot improve your outer life until you improve your inner life. If you have negative thoughts, negative actions will follow. If there is a chaotic mind, there will be chaos in one's life. In order to have a positive life and health, there must be positive thoughts. Based upon this belief I consider mental and spiritual aspects of health as important as physical health.

Thus, these are an important part of my program to remain healthy and prevent a recurrence. These include meditation, relaxation exercises, creative imagery, replacing negative with positive emotions, optimism, and affirmations among others. The processes of carrying out these exercises are presented in Chapter 10.

Meditation

I have consistently meditated for at least 30 minutes daily and usually in the evening or before I go to bed. For the past 6 years I have returned to a Search for God Group after being away for about 8 years and meditate with the group once a week at our meetings. Otherwise, I meditate alone. Efforts to get the group to set a time to meditate together in our own homes have been unsuccessful. At the end of each meditation I previously remembered those who needed prayers by calling out their names. More recently as the list gets longer and longer I have used a prayer box in which I place names of those requesting prayers. The names are obtained from several sources. Some are friends or family members needing prayers. Some are individuals who contact me because of their cancer prognosis and their desire to try alternative treatments. Others in my prayer box are individuals requesting prayers through social media sites such as Facebook.

I always pray for others at the end of my meditation when there is an increase in energy flow through me to send out to others. This is in accordance with the Edgar Cayce readings that were my foundation for many of my spiritual practices.

Relaxation

I usually carry out short relaxation exercises prior to meditation in the evening. These include some head and neck exercises, deep breathing, and brief relaxation that are discussed in Chapter 10.

Creative Imagery or Visualization and Thought Stopping

I do not use visualization or thought-stopping regularly but only occasionally when I have minor changes in my health condition or lifestyle. At those times I visualize a health outcome by using the process identified in Chapter 10.

Continual Positive Thoughts

I fill my mind with so many positive thoughts that there is no room for negative ones. I have done this successfully for many years and it is amazing. When I wake in the morning I think, "What a wonderful day – I feel so great today – I look forward to working on my radio program, or to writing or to talking with others for my radio show." I reinforce positive thoughts throughout the day and if I have a negative one, I immediately replace it with a positive one. For example, when someone cuts in front of me in his/her car on the highway I bless him/her and wish him/her a safe and happy day. Affirmations may be useful in this process of staying positive and replacing negative thoughts with positive ones and I have found that after being usually positive for years my health is great, and there are such good things in my life. *I Challenge You To Try This.*

Optimism – Remaining Positive

Closely related to remaining positive and changing negative thoughts to positive ones is optimism. I have found optimism is a great side effect of being positive and one that played a major role in staying healthy.

Optimism has been shown to be effective in increasing health and preventing illness. Earlier I presented a story of my mother's experience with cancer of the cervix of the uterus and how her optimism allowed her another 40 years of life post treatment. Optimism and a positive outlook were also a part of my treatment when I was diagnosed with lung cancer in 1974 and continue to the present day. One organization that assists individuals to develop an optimistic outlook is the Optimist Club. Their philosophy tells us a lot about how to develop optimism. Basically it involves having faith in ourselves, in God, and in others. Many of the spiritual and mental exercises discussed in this section have helped me to remain optimistic.

Affirmations

I have continually used affirmations since being free of cancer and these pertain to all aspects of my life including relationships, health, finances or whatever is of concern at the time. When I have had minor illnesses I have used affirmations of being healthy and well. When I retired and needed to move from the house where I lived I used affirmations that helped me find the right house to move to.

When I get bored with retirement and want something to do, I again use an affirmation until the desired outcome manifested. I usually have a few I am using at any one time. I do my affirmations when I walk the beach early each morning. There are few people on the beach at that time but if I see someone I stop so they do not think I am talking to myself even though I am actually talking to my unconscious mind, my higher self and sometimes God. Anne Marie Evers in her *Affirmations: Your Passport to Happiness* (2005) says affirmations when done properly always work and I have found that to be true.

Stress Reduction

Stress is a factor of life and helps to keep us motivated and growing. However, too much stress is detrimental to health. I view stress reduction as a holistic process including mental, physical and spiritual components. I use this process occasionally when I feel very stressed and I have developed techniques to help myself and others faced with stressful situations. In addition to information on stress reduction techniques discussed in Chapter 10, I have an ebook and a CD on stress and stress reduction available on my website for the interested reader.

Spiritual Aspects

I believe my spiritual activities are as important as my physical and mental activities in remaining well. These involve praying for others, working with spiritual attributes such as patience, love and forgiveness, and being of service to others. Exercises to strengthen these behaviors are presented in Chapter 10 and some that I use regularly will be discussed here.

Prayer for Self and Others

I hold daily prayers for those who are sick or have life problems and have asked for prayer. Prayers for self and others are held at the end of my daily meditation. Many people are familiar with prayers of petition in which we ask for something such as health for a loved one or a new job or lover. These are a part of my daily prayers. But there are other important types of prayer that I use depending upon the circumstances. I often give prayers of thanksgiving for the many blessings in my life and those in the lives of others for whom I pray and this helps me appreciate what I have. This also helps me build faith. For example, I may thank God for my health, home, friends, work, family and others. Despite changes in life circumstances I always find there are things to be thankful for.

Throughout life I have found that I sometimes pray for something and when it materializes I have forgotten about it and moved on to something else. Thus, now I must truly want something before I consider praying for it. At those times I have found that affirmations in combination with prayers work well for me. However, I also believe the desired outcome of the prayer must be in my best interest and I usually add, "for the good of all parties concerned," or "If it be thy will, Oh Lord. Bring only the best to me and others."

Occasionally I use confessional prayers in which I ask for forgiveness for some real or imagined wrongdoing. I may also talk with God about my feelings, attitudes, and problems so that I feel acceptance and can move on in life.

Faith

Faith was important when I had lung cancer and remains important as part of my daily activities for remaining cancer free. Faith is the "confident assurance that something we want is going to happen. It is the certainty that what we hope for is waiting for us, even though we cannot see it up ahead" (The Living Bible, Paraphrased, 1973). The story of Noah in the Bible is an example of faith. When Noah heard God's warning, he believed it even though there were no signs of flooding. Based upon this belief, Noah built a raft and saved his family.

Sometimes I do not get what I think I want at the moment. I then know that God has something better in mind for me and that eventually it will unfold. That is also faith. I have experienced this enough in life to know it to be true.

For me, faith relates to God, to myself and to my fellow man and I try to express my faith accordingly. The opposite of faith is doubt and when I doubt myself I doubt the God within. When I doubt my fellow man, I am not looking for the best in him/her that should be my ideal. Doubt is closely related to the negative feelings of fear and worry, and worry is a result of fear. And fear, in turn, is a result of doubt. The opposite of doubt is faith and for me faith is an important aspect of my life. In Luke 12:22–25 the Bible says, "What is the use of worrying? What good does it do? Will it add a single day to your life? No it will not. And if worry can't do such little things as that, what's the use of worrying about the bigger things."

It is difficult to not get caught up in doubt and fear in today's world where there is so much emphasis on negative things such as a terrorist attack, contaminated foods, global warming, food shortages, national deficit and on and on. It is this sensationalism that sells papers and brings people to the news on radio and television. But by working with the exercises presented in Chapter 10 I have adjusted my lifestyle so I rarely get caught up in this negativity. I do what I can do in such situations and then turn it over to God. For example, if I am confronted by a fearful situation I problem solve holistically to resolve the problem. For example, in relation to a potential attack, have I done all I can in the physical? Have I learned what to do in an emergency? Do I advocate with my government for the resources to protect the population? Are there other things I should do in the physical realm? Have I developed my faith? Have I used positive affirmations? Do I meditate for peace in the world? If I have done these, then I put my trust in God and replace fear with faith.

In addition, I remove negativity from my life as much as possible. If I watch the news knowing it will be mostly negative, I watch it only early in the day and never close to bedtime where it may affect my sleep and dream time. I almost never watch television and only listen to classical music on the radio. I avoid negative people as much as possible and search out positive people as friends and colleagues. I also find that as I have become more positive over the past 36 years I have attracted more and more positive people into my circle of friends and those who tended toward being negative have drifted away.

Forgiveness

Forgiveness not only improves relationships it also improves health. I have learned that carrying a grudge puts a weight on my shoulders and chest. From many years in A Search for God groups developing faith, patience, love and other attributes I have learned to accept behavior different from my own so that I rarely need to backtrack and forgive someone. However, when it is necessary I have used the exercises presented in Chapter 10 and hope they will be useful to you.

Service to Others

Jesus advocated being of service to others. This spiritual practice improves health when positive spiritual ideals and motives are underlying this service. Service to others may be separated into: 1) community services that emphasize service to groups; and 2) service to others that emphasize daily service to individuals. Exercises to strengthen both are presented in Chapter 10. I believe it is the little things in life that are important in our service to others whether it is a smile at a stranger, helping someone find their lost cat, sending a birthday card to a friend, or making a cake for his/her birthday. I am reminded of a friend who is a waitress and who says she likes her job because it allows her to talk with and be of service to others. She is always talking with her customers, offering comfort, patting them on the back for a job well done and other behaviors that shows that she truly cares about herself, others, and God. This to me is service to others. If this is not your usual pattern of behavior, try it. It will make you feel great.

Environment, Relationships and Politics
Environment

Environmental interventions are also necessary to remain cancer free. I am very aware of toxins in my environment and avoid these as much as possible so as not to overwhelm my immune system. Several strategies were mentioned earlier in this chapter including: 1) A diet of primarily organic foods to avoid toxins, pesticides, growth hormones, genetic engineering and others; 2) Eating primarily fruit, vegetables, nuts, grains and some seafood, fish and chicken; a minimal amount of pork. pasta, bread and other starches; no sugar, beef or fast foods. 3) Using supplements to strengthen diet and the immune system. 4) Use water that is deionized or spring water. 5) Using periodic detoxing to reduce the threat to the immune system. And 6) Avoidance of cigarette and tobacco smoke.

Other environmental interventions necessary for me and others who have had lung cancer include: 1) Avoidance of asbestos and radon at home or work. 2) Maintenance of a clean home environment free of dust, and other toxic substances. 3) Buy upholstered furniture, drapes and other items that do not give off toxins. 4) Allow no smoking in my home and avoiding any restaurants or other places where smoking is allowed. 5) Placed smoking and carbon monoxide detectors in strategic places at home; and replace batteries periodically. 6) Open windows to air my house when the weather allows and remove any toxins, smells or stale air. 7) Always open garage door before starting my car to avoid carbon monoxide fumes. 8) Supplements during the winter months such as Host Defense to strengthen the immune system in order to avoid pneumonia or other lung problems. 9) Remain indoors as much as possible when the air quality is poor. 10) Avoid the use of pesticides, herbicides and other lung and soil contaminants around my house. And 11) test for and remove radon under your house, if present.

Relationships

Maintaining relationships are also important in preventing a recurrence of lung cancer. This involved maintaining existing relationships and building new ones. Some techniques that I used for accomplishing this and research on its value are presented in Chapter 10.

Politics

I believe that being active in the political process is also an important part of life after cancer. For me this meant collecting for cancer organizations, contacting my congressman about pending legislation affecting cancer patients, writing letters to the editor and other activities that would further appropriate treatment for my fellow man. This is another way of giving back to the community. Techniques for several ways to work within the political process are discussed in Chapter 10.

Summary

In this chapter I have discussed things I have done over the past 36 years to prevent a recurrence of cancer. I reemphasize that for me a holistic approach was important and I worked with the physical, mental, spiritual aspects of my life as well as relationships, the environment and politics. At different times, some activities will take precedence over others but all are important.

Part III

Medical Aspects – Alternative
Interventions of Lung Cancer

Chapter 4

Alternative Medical Treatment at the Oasis Of Hope: Irt-C For Advanced Lung Cancer – Francisco Contreras, MD

Introduction

Lung cancer is still the leading cause of cancer death worldwide, reflecting the fact that it afflicts both sexes; it is estimated that 1.3 million people died of lung cancer in 2004. Most patients who develop this cancer are or have been chronic smokers, but up to 15% of cases are found in non-smokers who presumably have been exposed to second-hand smoke or other lung toxins such as radon, asbestos, or smog. The most common types of this cancer – so-called non-small cell cancers – are generally poorly responsive to chemotherapy and radiation – implying that cure is dependent on prompt and definitive surgery. Sadly, in a high proportion of cases, the cancer has spread beyond the possibility of surgical cure by the time the cancer is diagnosed.

Because advanced lung cancer is usually poorly or only transiently responsive to chemo- or radiotherapies, novel thera-peutic strategies are clearly needed for the many thousands of patients afflicted with this disorder. A promising approach in this regard is offered by the IRT-C protocol employed at Oasis of Hope Hospital (Tijuana, Mexico). In order to understand this therapy, you need to know something about a phenomenon known as 'oxidative stress'.

Oxidative Stress

The normal metabolism of living cells generates various metabo-lites of molecular oxygen that are known as 'reactive oxygen species' (ROS). These arise when a single electron is donated to molecular oxygen to generate the compound super oxide. The further metabolism of super oxide gives rise to highly reactive compounds such as hydrogen peroxide, hydroxyl radical, and peroxynitrite. An excess of these reactive compounds is known as 'oxidative stress', and can kill or severely damage cells. That's why all cells express a range of 'antioxidant' enzymes, which either convert these reactive compounds to harmless metabolites, or reverse their harmful structural effects.

Surprisingly, *moderate* levels of ROS actually can promote the proliferation of cells by boosting signaling by various growth factors. Indeed, many cancer cells are characterized by a chronic moderate production of ROS that actually increases their proliferation and survival, and makes them behave more aggressively, eating through neighboring healthy tissues and spreading to distant organs (metastasis) (Irani, K et al, 1998; Suh, Y et al, 1999; Brar, SS et al, 2002; Vaquero, EC et al, 2004; Dong, JM et al, 2004; Arnold, RS et al, 2001). This possibly explains why a high proportion of tumors express decreased levels of certain antioxidant enzymes – most notably, the enzyme catalase, which eliminates hydrogen peroxide (Sun, Y, 1990; Sun, Y et al, 1993; Rabilloud et al, 1990; Kwei, KA et al, 2004; Policastro, L et al, 2004).

This reduction in antioxidant activity promotes a modest increase in ROS levels that is often favorable to cancer growth, spread, and survival.

Using Oxidative Stress Theory in Lung Cancer Interventions

However, some insightful cancer scientists have grasped the fact that the relatively deficient antioxidant defenses in many tumors can be exploited as an 'Achilles heel'. These tumors should be relatively defenseless if a marked increase in ROS production within tumors can be achieved. And, remarkably, there is a very simple way to do this. In concentrations many fold higher than those ordinarily observed in the blood, vitamin C (aka ascorbate) can donate an electron to molecular oxygen to generate hydrogen peroxide (Chen, Q et al, 2005; Chen, Q et al, 2007). In normal healthy tissues, which possess ample levels of antioxidant enzymes such as catalase, this hydrogen peroxide is readily metabolized without harm to cells. But cancer cells can be much more vulnerable. Thus, researchers working with Dr. Mark Levine at the National Institutes of Health have shown that, in 5 of 9 cancer cell lines tested in culture, a one hour exposure to 5 mM ascorbate (equivalent to the concentration of glucose in the blood) killed at least 50% of the cells – whereas cell lines derived from healthy tissues tolerated 4 times this concentration without overt toxicity (Chen, Q et al, 2005).

Comparable concentrations of ascorbate can be achieved in tumors by intravenous infusion of sodium ascorbate in massive doses (Chen, Q, et al, 2007; Padayatty, SJ et al 2004). Indeed, the initial Linus Pauling protocol for vitamin C therapy of cancer included 10 days of high-dose intravenous vitamin C (Cameron, E et al, 1976). More recently, pioneering doctors such as Hugh Riordan have employed high-dose ascorbate infusions in cancer therapy, reporting objective remissions in some favorable cases (Rioran, HD et al, 2005; Padayatty, SJ et al, 2006). In addition, Dr. Mark Levine and colleagues have demonstrated that this strategy can retard cancer growth in mice (Chen, Q et al, 2008).

IRT-C Protocol at the Oasis of Hope

For several years, cancer doctors at Oasis of Hope Hospital have been using an 'IRT-C' protocol that involves intravenous adminis-tration of very high doses of sodium ascorbate. A dose of 30 grams is given during the first 30 minutes; after waiting for a further 90 minutes, a 'booster' dose of 30 grams is given (again over 30 minutes) to maintain the achieved elevation of tissue ascorbate levels. The intent of this regimen is to maintain potentially cytotoxic concentrations of ascorbate in the tumor for at least 4 consecutive hours (Padayatty, SJ et al, 2004). This regimen is very well tolerated, with no evidence of damage to healthy tissues. The only significant side effect is thirst – reflecting the fact that high-dose ascorbate exerts a diuretic effect (increased water loss through the kidneys). This is readily managed simply by giving the patient plenty of water to drink. It should be emphasized that, owing to inefficient absorption, *no amount* of *oral* vitamin C can achieve cytotoxic concentrations of ascorbate in tumors – which explains why clinical studies evaluating oral vitamin C in cancer therapy have had disappointing outcomes (Padayatty, SJ et al, 2004; Moertel, CO et al, 1985; Padayatty, SJ et al, 2000).

But the Oasis of Hope IRT-C protocol also employs several novel adjuvant measures intended to boost production of hydrogen peroxide in the tumor. The transfer of electrons from ascorbate to molecular oxygen within tumors is dependent on certain poorly-characterized metal-binding proteins which catalyze this transfer (Chen, Q et al, 2007); conceivably, the availability of these proteins could be rate-limiting for tumor hydrogen peroxide production. However, a type of vitamin K known as menadione is also highly effective for catalyzing hydrogen peroxide production by ascorbate (Calderon, PB et al, 2002; Verrax, L et al, 2005). Indeed, Belgian researchers have shown that menadione boosts the capacity of ascorbate to kill cancer cells in culture, and that co-administration of menadione amplifies the ability of high-dose vitamin C injections to control tumor growth in rodents (Calderon, PB et al, 2002; Gilloteaux, J, et al, 1998; Verrax, J et al, 2004; Verrax, J et al, 2006). So, to take advantage of this promising possibility, the Oasis of Hope IRT-C protocol also includes intravenous administration of a well-tolerated dose of menadione, given just a few minutes before the ascorbate infusion commences.

Another factor that is likely to be rate limiting for hydrogen peroxide production in ascorbate-treated tumors is oxygen (O_2) availability. It is well-known that many tumors have regions in which oxygen levels are very low, owing to fact that most tumors have a haphazard blood supply. It stands to reason that, during ascorbate therapy, these 'hypoxic' tumor regions will not be able to generate super oxide as rapidly as better-oxygenated regions. The Oasis of Hope IRT-C protocol therefore employs a couple of adjuvant measures intended to boost tumor oxygenation. One of these is a 'perfluorocarbon' oxygen-carrier molecule known as 'Perftec' (Verdin-Velasquez, RC et al, 2006). This was originally developed in Russia – under the name 'Perftoran'; when infused intravenously, it greatly enhances the oxygen-carrying capacity of blood, and thus can promote increased delivery of oxygen to hypoxic tumor regions. Having the patient inhale enriched oxygen in this regard further boosts the efficacy of Perftec. Also, on the day prior to ascorbate infusion, cancer patients are given a treatment – long popular in Europe – known as ozone autohemotherapy, which alters the properties of blood so that it is less viscous, its red blood cells are more flexible, and its oxygenated red blood cells surrender oxygen to tissues more readily (rightward shift of dissociation curve). Also, it promotes vasodilation by stimulating nitric oxide release by the endothelial lining of small arteries (Giunta, R et al, 2001; Bocci, V et al, 2005). The net result is more oxygen delivery to the tumor.

At-Home Regime for Oasis of Hope
Lung Cancer Patients

These are the key components of the IRT-C protocol. However, Oasis of Hope cancer patients also receive an elaborate 'at-home' regimen of nutraceuticals and safe drugs that are intended to slow cancer growth, support immune defense mechanisms, and reduce risk for certain common complications in cancer patients. This regimen includes agents such as high-dose vitamin D, selenium, silymarin, green tea extract, and the hormone melatonin. Remarkably, one of the strategies employed here is to *minimize* oxidative stress in the cancer, by administering high doses of an edible food algae, spirulina. Recent research shows that the chief phytonutrient in spirulina can potently inhibit an enzyme complex (NADPH oxidase) that generates much of the oxidative stress in many cancers (McCarty, MF, 2007a; McCarty, MF, 2007b). A reduction in oxidative stress can be expected to slow the proliferation and spread of many tumors. Thus, we have described our IRT-C regimen as a 'two-phase' protocol in which we intermittently subject tumors to extreme, potentially lethal oxidative stress, while at other times minimizing oxidative stress in tumors to slow their growth (McCarty, MF, 2007b).

Comparison of Survival Rates: Oasis of Hope and Conventional

Lung cancers that have spread beyond the point of surgical cure are obvious candidates for IRT-C, particularly since most lung cancers are poorly responsive to chemotherapy. In 2011, we concluded a 5 year prospective study utilizing IRT-C with stage four lung cancer patients. We have survival rates for years 1 through 5. We can compare our results with comparable survival rates for stage 4 lung cancer reported by the National Cancer Institute's SEER Program, which determines average survivals for cancer patients in many regions of the US (National Cancer Institute, 2007). Here's how the Oasis of Hope IRT-C survival rates compare with those of conventional therapy.

As you can readily see in the figure (page 98), our patients with advanced lung cancer receiving IRT-C tend to survive much longer than those treated in the US. Comparing IRT-C with conventional therapy, 1-year survivals were 82% vs. 20%; 2-year survivals 50% vs. 6%; 3-year survivals 27% vs. 3%; 4-year survivals 23% vs. 2%; and 5-year survivals 9% vs. 1.6% At the conclusion of our clinical study, results with IRT-C were nearly 6 times better than the results using conventional therapy.

While we are very encouraged by this, it is evident that we are

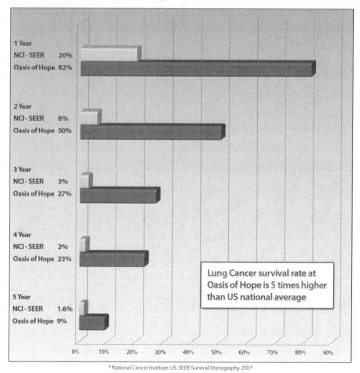

Figure 4.1

still a long way away from our ultimate goal of turning advanced cancer into a disease that can be managed chronically like diabetes – for decades if need be. We have therefore undertaken some additional initiatives that should be able to improve our therapeutic outcomes. In particular, we recently have introduced a novel form of cancer immunotherapy – allergenic lymphocyte immunotherapy – first successfully employed in Japan over 25 years ago, but largely ignored by the cancer research establishment until recently (Kondo, M, et al, 1984; Symons, HJ, et al, 2008; Su X, Guo, S et al, 2009). This well-tolerated strategy appears to have the potential to induce objective tumor regression in a substantial minority of cancer patients; we therefore suspect that, when employed in conjunction with IRT-C, it likely will improve long-term therapy outcomes.

We are also revising our treatment plans so that patients will be encouraged to return to Oasis of Hope more frequently for booster courses of IRT-C. It stands to reason that, in patients with responsive tumors, a more frequent application of ascorbate therapy should achieve better cancer control.

Finally, we are considering additional adjuvant strategies that might further enhance oxidative stress in ascorbate-treated tumors. In a recently published scientific paper, we propose that measures which concurrently deprive tumor cells of glucose should amplify oxidative stress in tumor cells by selectively impairing their antioxidant defenses (McCarty, MF, 2010). In the future, we hope to evaluate this option in experimental treatment protocols.

Case Study of YG – Age 68
Diagnosis: Stage IV Adenocarcinoma of the Lung

This female patient was diagnosed in March of 2007 with primary adenocarcinoma of the lung with metastasis to the bones and contra-lateral lung according to a PET scan taken April 24, 2007. The patient also was diagnosed with emphysema and chronic bronchitis. She was offered chemotherapy, which she refused.

She came to the Oasis of Hope on April 24, 2007 in good general condition without respiratory distress but significant left shoulder pain. She began Integrative Regulatory Therapy with high-dose vitamin C. She was discharged May 10, 2007 and a CT scan showed that the primary tumor and metastasis had not grown and the patient's quality of life improved significantly but the pain cause by a metastasis to the third left rib was still quite painful. We recommended palliative radiation therapy, which she received once she returned to South Africa, her home.

On July 24, 2007, a follow-up visit to Oasis, we took a new CT scan that reported stable tumor activity. Outside of her usual emphysema and bronchitis symptoms, the patient reported good quality of life and she stopped all analgesics. Continues with our IRT-C program.

A follow-up PET scan from South Africa on February 6, 2008 reported she had stable disease, No new lesions were seen. She continues with our IRT-C program.

On her follow-up visit to Oasis of Hope on November 3, 2008, a new CT scan shows significant improvement of the primary lesion and rib metastasis and no change of the contra-lateral metastasis. The patient has excellent quality of life and continues with our IRT-C program.

Another follow-up PET scan from South Africa on February 12, 2009 reports relative increase of the primary lesion but otherwise stable disease. No new lesions were seen. She continues with our IRT-C program.

Another follow-up visit to Oasis of Hope on October 26, 2009 showed she was clinically stable and in good to excellent quality of life. She continues with our IRT-C program.

The patient to date is in excellent condition and her stage IV lung cancer is stable.

Summary

This chapter has focused on the medical protocol that we have developed and utilized successfully over the years to help patients suffering from stage IV lung cancer. On our website, www.oasisofhope.com, you will find out about our treatment philosophy and the context in which our therapies are provided. Oasis of Hope was established in 1963 with the purposes of caring for the whole person: body, mind and spirit; sharing the healing power of faith hope and love; and advancing science and medicine to put an end to cancer one patient at a time. Our IRT-C treatment program is one of the many fruits produced over five decades of treating patients with advanced stages of cancers.

Chapter 5

Alternative Medical Treatment – Lung Cancer: At the Cancer Screening and Treatment Center of Nevada and Century Wellness Clinic – James Forsythe, MD, HMD

Introduction

Cancer is the leading cause of death from any illness or disease in patients under 80 years of age. There are approximately 1.5 million new cases of cancer from any source in the United States yearly, and lung cancer, long being the number one killer from cancers in men in the past years, has become the number one killer in women, surpassing breast cancer previously in that position.

In 2010 there is predicted to be 84,000 deaths in men, representing 31% of all male cancers. There is also predicted to be 71,000 deaths in women, representing 26% of all female cancers. In fact, lung cancer causes more deaths than breast, colon and prostate cancer combined.

As is true in all cancers, the survival rate is directly proportional to the presenting stage at diagnosis. In non-small cell lung cancer approximately 24% of the patients are diagnosed in the earliest/stage I disease state and have a survival rate of approximately 70% at five years, whereas a more advanced, stage III lung cancer carries an average survival rate of 30% at five years.

Conventional Lung Cancer Treatments and Survival

Modern conventional lung cancer studies are now looking into predictive biomarkers to determine which drugs may be most effective in non-small cell lung cancer. In general, low levels of these genetic biomarkers correlate with increased sensitivity to certain standard drug specific protocols containing Platinum, Taxane, Gemcitabine, Pemetrexed and Erlotinib.

As an example, low levels of genetic biomarkers RRMI and ERCC would best be treated by the combination of CisPlatinum and Gemzar. Another example would be a positive KRAS mutation, indicating an expected benefit from the use of the targeted therapy Erbitux.

The new and emerging super-subspecialty of Integrative Oncology has evolved in large part due to the dismal failure and negligible benefits of long-term or greater than 5 years of chemotherapy in adults with stage IV cancers, which, as reported by the *Journal of Clinical Oncology* in 2004, indicated in a large retrospective study, which was compared with a similar Australian study, only a 2.1% overall survival rate in the United States compared to a 2.3% survival rate in Australia. Both results were clinically statistically similar.

Outcome-based studies in the United States using integrative protocols, have recently shown results over a five-year period in adult stage IV cancers with a 20-fold increase in survival rate compared to these extremely poor conventional results. No simple investigative new drug application given to the FDA would pass muster or be approved with this incredibly low response rate.

A patient today diagnosed with stage III and IV non-small cell lung cancer could be prescribed at any large cancer center the drug Cisplatinum and Taxol. This combination is based strictly on prospective clinical studies, showing that this duo has the best overall response rate. A close second to this combination would be Cisplatin and Gemzar.

If the patients has advanced disease, a targeted therapy such as Avastin, which inhibits angiogenesis, or an epithelial growth factor receptor could be added as a third drug.

It is important to remember that lung cancers are divided into two major sub-classes: 1) small cell carcinomas; and 2) non-small cell carcinomas. Under the category of small cell carcinoma there is only one single histological group, and that is the small cell carcinoma. However, there are four major types of non-small cell carcinomas, including: 1) large cell carcinoma; 2) squamous cell carcinoma; 3) bronchioalveolar; and 4) adenocarcinoma. Some classifications will include mesotheliomas as a firth type. Mesotheliomas are, strictly speaking, a tumor originating on the surface of the lung or lining the pleural cavity.

If the patient is an Asian, female, non-smoker, the targeted oral therapy, named 'Tarceva' is often added either in combination or as a single agent. A typical second and third-line protocol for non-small lung cancer in stages III and IV would be: 1) Carboplatinum + Navelbine; or 2) Pemetrexed. Either of these protocols could add the targeted therapies of either Avastin or Srbitux. A reasonable, and often used, third-line protocol would be: 1) Carboplatin and VP-16; or 2) Taxotere and Avastin.

Small cell carcinomas have a propensity to metastasize early and often spread to the central nervous system so that radiation therapy is rarely used except in the very early, Stage I disease; whereas, chemotherapy is more often used in all of the late stages.

A typical first-line treatment with small cell carcinomas would include: Adriamycin + Cytoxan + VP-16, or Methotrexate + Vincristine + Cytoxan + Adriamycin.

A second-line protocol for small cell carcinomas would likely be a combination of IFEX/Mesna/Carboplatin/VP-16, and a reasonable third-line protocol might consist of Carboplatinum and Gemzar.

Any time an oncologist reaches a third, fourth or fifth-line treatment protocol this becomes 'off-label' usage and is not considered 'evidence-based medicine' but rather judgment-based or simply stated 'practicing the art of medicine'.

Integrative Medicine

Because Integrative Medicine was never taught or mentioned in medical school curricula until the late 1990s, this has caused most physicians and even patients to complain that, "If this type of medicine worked, why is it not taught in medial school and why don't most doctors use this discipline?"

Unfortunately, political and economic forces within the United States and other countries actively suppress news favorable to alternative treatments. This is because 'Big Pharma', the FDA, the NIH, and the NCI will not allow changes in this malfunctioning system because of the financial rewards that are present by keeping the status quo.

In fact, most conventional oncologists are oblivious to the fact that the politics and economics of cancer medicine trump the science of cancer medicine. In addition, they seem to be ignorant or uncaring to the long-term poor results from prolonged chemotherapy and the multiple chronic toxicities which they cause, which only serves to damage the quality of life and also the immune system of those who survive.

While there has never been a 'panacea' or 'magic bullet' yet developed to treat cancer, and there is no cancer yet to respond 100% to any single drug or group of drugs in any protocol, the successful oncologist of the future must address the whole person, their emotional profile, their nutritional needs, their supplemental needs, the detoxification of their underlying heavy-metal and chemical toxins, the integrity of their immune system, their dental health, and most of all serving to protect their entire anatomical, physiological and biochemical system from undue toxicity and excessive amounts of radiation, surgery and massive doses of chemotherapy. The onslaught of these factors leaves the bodies intrinsic defense mechanisms, immune function, white cells, natural killer cells, and B & T cells all totally depleted.

In the last 50 years statistics have shown that the number of new cases of cancers have steadily increased. In comparison with other diseases such as cardiovascular diseases and infectious diseases like influenza and pneumonia, there has been a poor overall response to cancer in any form. In fact, the death rate from all types of cancer within the last 50 years has only decreased by 5%, whereas with other diseases there has been a 50% to 60% decrease in death rates.

Since 1971 and over 100-billion dollars later, when President Richard M. Nixon announced his goal to conquer cancer, symbolized by his 'war on cancer', there has been a steady increase in cancer cases diagnosed in the United States, and today this number approaches 1.5 million cases per year and overall 560,000 deaths per year in 2010. In the end, the steady increase in cancer deaths over the past 39 years, since the 'war on cancer' was begun, this must mute any claims of victory by anyone fighting the 'war on cancer'.

Integrative Oncology, which treats the whole body and the whole person, looks more into the self-healing properties of the body as well as the molecular biology of the cancer cell itself, including the importance of sugar-free diets, alkalinizing diets, bio-oxidative therapies, specific vitamin supplemental therapies, herbal therapies, amino acid supplements, as well as the all important energetics of the cancer itself. The use of these modalities along with low-dose fractionated chemotherapy or insulin potentiating therapies in combination with immune stimulating and supportive therapies will in the long run contribute to a higher success rate and less side-effects with less toxic burden on the human system. Along with this the use of chemosensitivity testing, which is all important to identify through genetic markers, the important and specific chemotherapy drugs that are useful to each specific patient's cancer, along with the over 50 different supplements which can be identified to be useful in an individual cancer case again based upon genetic markers.

Symptoms of Lung Cancer and Diagnostic Process

The common symptoms of lung cancer include a cough that does not go away or lingers long after an episode of sinusitis, upper respiratory infection or bronchitis has ended. The cough tends to persist and the sputum may be colored (yellow, green, brown or bloody), and multiple courses of antibiotics often times have no effect on reducing the duration or intensity of the cough. There may also be early weight loss and anorexia. There may be pleuritic chest pain, which is pain that is evoked by deep breathing, which is lancinating and often painful on one side of the chest or the other. There may be signs and symptoms of metastases from the lung cancer, which may precede the actual diagnosis.

These could be in the form of central nervous system symptoms such as headaches, dizziness, motor or sensory loss, or seizures related to brain metastases. There may be bone pain in any bone of the body where metastases have caused destruction of bony matrix. There may be fluid buildup in the lung, which impedes breathing and causes increased shortness of breath, and is a result of malignant pleural effusions, which may fill up either side of the lung and make it difficult for the patient to sleep on the non-effected side.

These symptoms will only cause the patient to seek medical attention with their personal family care physician or internist, and most likely the patient will be placed on a cough medicine or possibly even on antibiotics in combination. If after one week, 10 days or even two weeks these symptoms do not abate, most likely a chest x-ray will be taken and the discovery of a mass on one side or the other of the lung, or possibly an effusion on one side of the lung or the other may be seen on the chest x-ray, along with some fullness of the mediastinum or central portion of the chest, possibly with an effusion around the heart or in the roots of the lung, so called 'hila'. There may be fullness or a distinct mass.

The most likely course of events following these findings

would cause the primary physician to direct the patient to a surgeon, radiologist or oncologist for further diagnostic maneuvers. These maneuvers would likely consist of a CAT scan of the chest and possibly a PET scan to determine if the suspected mass or above findings are related to cancer. Additionally, important tumor markers for lung cancer, including the CEA or CA19-9, would be useful to verify the presence of a malignant condition.

After the numbing details of your work-up have been discussed by your chosen oncologist or surgeon, and after a biopsy has been performed via either a needle biopsy of the lung, a pleural biopsy of the pleural fluid, or a mediastinal biopsy, or the findings after bronchoscopy with biopsy of suspicious lesions of the tracheobronchial tree, a pathologic diagnosis will be made which will define the cancer as being that of either a small cell or a cancer of the non-small cell origin. As discussed earlier in this chapter, the non-small cell varieties are more common and would include adenocarcinoma, large cell carcinoma, squamous cell carcinoma, or bronchioalveolar cancer.

After the details of the pathological diagnosis have been discussed with the patient by their chosen primary care physician, the referring oncologist or referring thoracic surgeon, the full force of conventional oncology kicks into overdrive. This, of course, refers to the modalities of surgery, radiation therapy, and chemotherapy, singly, doubly or in triplicate.

Rarely if ever does a meaningful discussion of secondary options for alternative treatment, including diet, nutrition, alkalinization, bio-oxidative therapies or supplementation occur. In fact, even if the patient approaches these subjects, they are generally disregarded by the physician with either a stern look or a categorical statement of negativity, much like "they are useless", "they will do no good", or "there is no evidence-based medicine behind any of these options". And finally, "if you choose to use anything but conventional therapy, you will have to find another oncologist".

All of these statements tell the patient either directly or indirectly that this particular physician is in charge of your care and they intend to keep it that way. He has demonstrated closed-mindedness to all alternative therapies.

At this point, if patients are aware of what is going on, they will tell themselves that if in fact they choose to seek a second opinion, and especially an Alternative Medicine opinion, they had better keep this information to themselves.

On the conventional side, for lung cancers which are in early stages, thoracic surgical consultation would be the first step in the treatment protocol, and if the tumor is isolated and is an early stage I, surgical removal of one or two, possible even up to three lobes of one lung would be removed, probably then followed by radiation therapy and chemotherapy. In stage IV lung cancer disease the desired conventional treatment would consist of surgical biopsy followed by chemotherapy, or just chemotherapy alone.

In difficult cases, or where there is some question regarding the sequence of therapy or the appropriateness of certain therapies, a tumor board will convene and the attending primary doctor, medical oncologist, or surgeon, or perhaps even the radiation therapist, or all of the above, will recommend that the tumor board review the case. These boards as a rule are run by the Pathology Department and usually include the involved surgeon or surgeons, the pathologist, the oncologist, the radiologist, and the referring primary care physicians, as well as another interested staff physicians.

While there is always hope for a unanimous opinion as to the proper course of treatment, very often there is no consensus of opinion and it is then left up to the referring physician or oncologist to make the final treatment decision. After the tumor board deliberation it may be the providence of the lone oncologist to prepare treatment protocol and present it to the patient. At this point the patient has an agonizing and difficult decision to make.

He may say to himself, "Am I doing the right thing?" "Should I seek a second opinion?" "Is it time to look for another option or opinion?" Or "Should I go to a large cancer center for another opinion or possibly just go on experimental treatment?"

Chemo Sensitivity Testing

It is important to realize at this point, especially in stage IV disease, that genetic chemosensitivity testing is absolutely essential in that it can precisely pinpoint the most specific drug or drugs necessary to treat the patient's specific condition. These tests are run in various parts of the world, including Greece, Germany and Korea. These tests are widely used in Central and South America, Europe and Asia.

The information obtained from these tests has a turn around time of anywhere from one to three weeks, but they are essential in that they provide a blueprint or road map to identify the best drugs and best supplements for each individual patient.

Without utilizing these modalities, conventional medical oncologists are basically 'shooting in the dark' and fooling themselves and the patients that they really know exactly what drugs are best for this particular patient and his cancer.

Typical Treatments by Integrative Physicians

It is at this point where most Integrative Oncologists, when sought out for a second or third opinion, will offer the following options:

- Strict protocol chemotherapy based on the results of chemosensitivity testing.
- Low-dose fractionated chemotherapy, either alone or with insulin potentiation.
- Either one or two of the above with complementary therapies, based on supplemental information from genetic marker testing.

- Complementary therapy alone, based on chemosensitivity testing.
- Best supportive therapy for patients who are too far advanced for any other type of treatment.

Among the high-tech chemosensitivity testing laboratories around the world, the Greek test known as the "Research Genetic Cancer Center Test" is the most advanced and evaluates 19 different families of chemotherapy agents, as well as 38 different supplements. Even hydrogen peroxide and hyperthermia are tested and scored for efficacy.

The chemosensitivity testing methodology includes the following:

- Isolation from cancer cells and development of primary cultures.
- Each culture includes in the cultivation media a cytostatic drug.
- Testing of genes by micro-array analysis which becomes targets for cytostatics, or they are involved in resistant phenotype, or they are involved in the metastatic procedure.
- Verification of the analysis by small scale viable testing of the cultures.

Like everything else in medicine, there are no absolutes and the Integrative Oncologist's judgment comes into play significantly in the production of the protocol, and this in reality is the practice of the 'art of medicine'.

Evidenced Based Testing and Results of Cancer Treatment At the Cancer Screening and Treatment Center of Nevada

Over the past twelve years, and some fourteen years after acquiring my Boards in Homeopathic Medicine, and passing the

Nevada State written and oral examinations, I embarked on a mission to research natural supplements in what is called 'outcome-based' studies. The major impetus for this decision was the prevalent opinion by conventional medicine that any type of alternative or complementary medicine was devoid and lacking in any scientific foundation or, in short, it was not 'evidence-based'.

As a famous professor of nutritional medicine at UCLA remarked at a large medical symposium held in Reno, Nevada: "Any time any patient is taking more than two separate drugs in their body, there is *no* 'evidence-based' medicine." Because pharmaceutical-supported clinical studies rarely test more than two drugs in the same individual at any one time, a patient taking three or more drugs loses all possibilities of being an 'evidence-based' subject.

Being an integrative oncologist, my colleagues and peers in medicine have looked at any natural therapies as being worthless or at least highly suspect for any efficacy.

In the late 1990s, I was asked by research scientists employed by Nature Sunshine out of Utah to conduct an 'outcome-based' study on the supplement "Paw Paw". This product is a chemical acetogenin from the twig of the paw paw tree, indigenous to the Southeastern United States. This product's main action is directed at the energetic properties of cancer cells which are inherently low-energy systems producing only five percent of the energy molecules AMP, ADP and ATP as a non-cancerous cell. Paw paw hyper-energizes the cancer cell to the degree that the cell cascades into apoptosis, or what is known in the industry as 'programmed cell death'.

One hundred patients were acquired in this study, all of whom were stage IV adult cancers of various origins. This study was carried out for three years and showed greater than 28% survival rates and no significant toxic profiles, or adverse reactions, other than mild gastrointestinal upsets including mild bloating and nausea in less than 25% of the patients. Today this product is used worldwide and is even being used to treat small animal cancers.

A second study was begun in 2004 on a product called "Poly-MVA". Developed by Dr. Merrill Garnet of the McKeen-Garnet Laboratories, located on Long Island, New York. This liquid supplement had undergone extensive animal studies since the 1980s and at the time of my study initiation was being used by over 800 medical doctors in over 30 countries throughout the world. Its main components were Palladium (a rare earth metal) and Alpha Lipoic Acid (ALA), which was tightly bound to the Palladium and mixed with a number of complementary vitamins, minerals and amino acids. The vitamins consisted of vitamin B1, vitamin B2 and vitamin B12. The amino acids consisted of Formyl-Methionine and N-Acetylcysteine. Several trace minerals were also added to the brew, and these are Rhodium and Ruthenium. The minerals were added to balance the pH and act as a catalyst for the chemical reactions. Conventional scientific and biochemical literature have reported that Palladium combined with alpha-lipoic acid had anticarcinogenic properties.

A key concept underlying the molecular behavior of Poly-MVA was the fact that cancer cells not only demand and thrive on simple sugars but that simple sugars must be 'fermented' or metabolized without oxygen in order for the cancer cells to produce life-sustaining energy in the form of ATP. The key enzyme in this process is Pyruvate Dehydrogenase, which is the connecting link between aerobic metabolism and anaerobic metabolism. Cancer cells are, by evolutionary design, low-energy systems and produce only five percent of the energy of a normal cell.

The unique pairing of Palladium with alpha-lipoic acid provides both the properties of electrochemical electron trans-ferring with the most powerful antioxidant and detoxifier known to the human body. This compound is both water and fat soluble, and as such is able to cross the often-impenetrable blood-brain barrier.

Alpha-lipoic acid is present in the intracellular energy factories called 'mitochondria' and helps neutralize free radicals, and it is vital to the activation of vitamins E, C, and glutathiones. Glutathione levels are low in all cancer patients.

The proven benefits of Poly-MVA include the following:

Aid in cellular energy production
Support hepatic function
Detoxify liver toxins
Improve neurologic functions
Chelate heavy metals
Improve blood formation components
Protect normal cells against free radical damage

The study, begun in 2004, accrued 225 patients and it has now continued to be followed with follow-up statistics over a six-year period of time. The study itself was questioned by the FDA, and during my ordeal with the FDA. with regard to my human growth hormone studies, they actually subpoenaed all of my patient charts without HIPPA authorization in order to verify the favorable results demonstrated by my 'outcome-based' study. In summary, the FDA found no fault with my research procedures or clinical studies, and no fault with my charting and follow-up parameters. As a consequence, no indictments regarding my Poly-MVA study were ever forthcoming from the FDA or the Federal prosecutors.

The results of this study, now over a five-year period, have shown over a 30% continued overall survivorship. This compares to conventional oncology's 2.1% one-year survival rate. The best responders in this study were those patients who were suffering from stage IV prostate or breast cancer or non-Hodgkin lymphomas.

Most Recent Evidence-Based Study and Results Compared to Conventional Oncology

In June of 2005, my third study I added a plant-based, natural homeopathic substance which was initiated with the sponsorship of a private company. This privately owned supplement company had reported anecdotal and surprisingly impressive results in cancer patients. However, they had not conducted any approved FDA clinical studies, and certainly nothing to convince conventional medicine or integrative medical oncology that these results were nothing more than spontaneous remissions or unexplained, meaningless statistical results.

This study was carried out on adult stage IV cancers of various origins. After five years, which culminated in August 2010, 500 patients were accrued. The overall response rate of all these patients, who had been on integrative cancer protocols, Forsythe Immune Therapy (FIT) has been calculated to be 46%. For lung cancer there were 65 patients with all forms of lung cancer with 19 patients demonstrating overall survival, or a 39%, five-year, ongoing 'outcome-based' study result. This result compares favorably with the conventional literature that shows that stage IV patients of all types are unlikely to have a survival rate of greater than five percent (5%).

Typical Case Study

A typical case history would be patient MS, a 52 year old, white female living in Carson City, Nevada, who was registered in this study in 2005 with stage IV non-small cell lung cancer, which had metastasized to her mediastinum and her other lung. She had been given between three and six months to live by her conventional doctors. She is alive today and on no chemotherapy at the present time, over five years later, in excellent health and fully active with a 100% performance status.

All Evidence-Based Studies Utilized Natural Substances

It should be noted that the results of all three of my studies, the Paw Paw study, the Poly-MVA study, and the current FIT study, were all done with natural substances which are homeopathically approved by the Nevada State Board of Homeopathic Medicine, and which were given to patients either with conventional chemotherapy or with low dose fractionated chemotherapy or with low dose insulin-potentiated therapy. Also these protocols were used with the addition of Poly-MVA as a separate supplement, or were given as a single agent. Therefore, all of the results involved the above separate options.

No Side Effects for Patients

All of the three studies showed no significant adverse toxicities, including no hair loss, nausea, vomiting or diarrhea, no skin rashes, no chemo-brain syndromes, no cardiac toxicity, no hepatic or renal toxicities, and no bone marrow suppression of any kind. There was also no evidence of any peripheral neuropathies nor any problems related to quality of life issues.

Chemosensitivity Testing

In the last two years of my final FIT study, from 2008 through the present time and ongoing, I have added a very valuable asset to the diagnostic workup of my patients with advanced stage IV lung cancer. This innovation, which is only being done throughout the United States by several other clinics, includes chemosensitivity testing at the German Biofocus Laboratories in Germany or the Greek Chemosensitivity Test, referred to as the Research Genetic Cancer Center in Florina, Greece. A new chemosensitivity laboratory is also being looked at in Korea called the Good gene Laboratories.

The Greek test (RGCC) has been especially helpful in giving the patients a blueprint or road map to not only the best drugs for their specific cancer which is derived by sending whole blood samples to Germany or Greece, or Korea for genetic analysis or 'decoding' and receiving (within a two-week period) a list of the exact drugs out of 18 families of chemotherapy agents, including targeted agents, and the best supplements, including a list of over 38 separate cancer active supplements, the best supplements which can be used to augment the effects of the drugs, either alone or in combination with the chemotherapy drugs, a protocol which would give the patient the most precise knowledge of which chemotherapy agents, which targeted agents and which hormones are best for their particular cancers, and also which supplements out of the list of 38 would best help the patient achieve a complete and more lasting response to therapy.

It is important to remember that when giving the wrong chemotherapy drugs, you are giving poison to the patient without benefit. However, when you give the wrong supplements this may not harm the patient in any way but it is certainly a drain on their financial capacities and it does not help in suppressing tumor growth.

Other Treatments at the Cancer Screening and Treatment Center of Nevada and Century Wellness Clinic

Our clinic also emphasizes looking for the source of the cancer through hair analysis and toxic metal evaluation, followed by chelation therapy, also looking at dental health, chemical toxicities, allergic considerations, nutritional considerations including a low, simple sugar diet, alkalinization and electrodermal testing to ferret out any internal organ imbalances.

Our clinic offers a three-week loading dose of the immune therapies, FIT along with intravenous Poly-MVA, or both in combination. During this three- week period patients are also given high-dose vitamin C infusions and hydrogen peroxide infusions, both of which are established treatment modalities with the Nevada State Board of Homeopathic Medicine.

Home Follow-Up Care

When patients are discharged from our clinic they are sent home with support supplements specific to their own individual cancers, and specific to the recommendations of the chemosensitivity testing laboratories. They are also sent home with protocols, either for conventional chemotherapy or low dose, non-toxic insulin potentiated therapies, as recommended by their chemosensitivity test results. Follow-up is via telephone or in a three-month period where patients return to our clinic for at least a one-week re-evaluation and booster treatment session. Overall, I would say that the chemosensitivity testing has been the most important addition to achieving excellent remission in my cancer patients.

Chapter 6

Mind-Body Medicine – Bernie Siegel, MD

Introduction

We all need to be aware that though our bodies experience many illnesses, which can threaten our lives, that our body loves us. The ability to heal and cure our bodies is built into our body. After I operate upon someone I do not need to give them instructions about how to heal their incision. The mechanisms are all present and the intelligence of the body knows what to do. However, if we do not enjoy our life and body our body has a lot harder time healing because of the internal chemistry created by the negative emotions and feelings. I can recall someone I operated upon for cancer. He was doing very well and I told him he could go home that day. To save him some time and effort after discharge I said we would have the oncologist see him before he left. I came back several hours later and he had a high fever due to an infected wound. I knew that the despair caused by the oncologist's words had made him vulnerable.

We must also understand that it is no accident that Monday morning has the highest incidence of heart attacks, strokes, illnesses and suicides. If we do not love our bodies and our lives our body's response is to use illness and death as a way to free us from the life we do not enjoy and desire. From our body's perspective death is not the worst outcome because it makes us perfect again free of our physical afflictions and limitations.

Our genes do not make decisions. They are stimulated by our internal chemistry to become active and either kill or cure. When actors are given a comedy to perform, and their blood is drawn while acting, immune function is enhanced and stress hormone levels decrease. The opposite happens when they are given a tragedy to perform. We are all actors, often just playing a role in our lives instead of living an authentic life, and must realize how our feelings affect our internal chemistry and health.

Influence of Personality on Health and Illness

Genes do not make the decisions, they are stimulated into activity by this internal chemistry. Identical twins do not get the same disease on the same day. Their personality plays an important part though they share genes. The twin who internalizes anger and tries to please everyone by doing what makes them happy is far more likely to develop breast cancer than her independent sister who is living her authentic life and expressing her feelings. There is survival behavior and an immune competent personality. It is not very complicated to define and studies show that our personalities relate to the diseases we develop and our ability to survive. One can predict from an individual's personality and drawings of herself what diseases are more likely to occur and where.

When one has meaning in one's life, expresses appropriate anger, asks for help from friends and family, says no to things they do not want to do, makes therapeutic decisions rather than having them imposed, takes time to play and enjoy life, uses feelings to make them aware of their needs just as hunger makes them seek nourishment and lives an authentic life and not a role or one imposed upon them, they are far more likely to be a survivor.

Successful Behavior and Self-Induced Healing

Doctors do not study success as much as they should. They are aware of successful treatments but often not about successful behavior. So if you get well when you are not supposed to you have a spontaneous remission or miracle. Neither of which teaches the doctor anything. But what if the doctor asked you, as I learned to do and observe: why didn't you die when you were supposed to? Then you would share your story and the doctor would learn something he or she could share with other patients. In his book *Cancer Ward*, Solzhenitsyn uses the term self-induced healing and describes it as a rainbow colored butterfly fluttering out of the book one of the men is reading and they all held up their foreheads and cheeks for its healing touch as it flew past. Self-induced healing is the term doctors should be talking about and learning how to perform it from their successful patients.

The key I learned was what the symbolism portrays. The rainbow represents all our emotions, each color represents a feeling as is displayed in the work I do with patient's drawings, and the butterfly is the symbol of transformation. So when does self-induced healing occur? When we transform our lives and create peace and order. Basically we are rebirthing ourselves and by being born again giving our body a new message, which leads it to strive to preserve our life and health. Years ago a retiring landscaper came to see me with cancer of the stomach. After surgery I told him he needed more treatment, as I couldn't remove all the cancer. He said, "You forgot something. It is springtime and I am going home to make the world beautiful before I die." To make a long story short he lived to age ninety-four with no sign of cancer. He spent his life devoted to making the world beautiful and his body got the message and partici-pated. Though he did develop a hernia "from lifting boulders in my landscape business" which I repaired. So don't ever retire but engage and disengage and keep your life interesting.

Visualization and Becoming

One more symbolic item: I mentioned the need to find peace and order but that can't be done until you quiet your mind and your life. For me the symbolism is in the image of the still pond. The ugly duckling is able to see he is a swan and a tiger, brought up by goats, sees he is really a tiger when they see their reflections in the still water. If they let memories of a painful past be what they focused upon they would never get to know their true selves. So quiet your life and mind and see your true reflection and life. Then you truly are born again into the true self and save your life by losing the life imposed upon you. You can also visualize becoming the person you want to become and eliminating any illness. I use the word eliminate versus kill because it is important for each person to use the image that feels right for them be it God's light melting a block of ice, which represents your tumor, a dog eating meat or a bird eating birdseed as your immune system. They all have worked for people.

What I constantly look for and prescribe are the common themes, which lead to rebirth. They can be found in the works of all kinds of survivors from members of the armed forces to recovering addicts. As AA teaches, fake it till you make it. So rehearse and practice becoming the person you want to be. Look for coaches and constructive criticism from all the people in your life. They can help to keep you on the track to a new self. I also recommend that you choose a new name for yourself as you embark on this journey.

Influence of Beliefs and Images on Treatment and Life Outcome

Our mind is a very powerful instrument and our beliefs and images play an important role in our response to treatment. A radiation therapist told me that he felt terrible because he just learned, while doing his routine monthly inspection of their machine, that after the machine was repaired no one put the radioactive cobalt back into it. So he hadn't treated anyone for a month. I told him he would have to be an idiot to not know he hadn't treated anyone so he had tumors shrinking and people having side effects because they thought they were being treated. He said, "Oh my God you're right."

So there are times a treatment works because you believe in it and not because the treatment itself is of any benefit. I tried to deceive people into health whenever I could. Especially children, whom I did surgery on, because I knew they believed in me. So I used my words in a therapeutic way. Wordswordsword become swordswordswords and we can kill or cure with a scalpel or a word. When hope is taken away by a doctor's predictions I have watched people go home and climb into bed and die. Also when we live a role and it ends, for example when men can't work anymore they die or when the kids all leave home momma dies because they now find 'no reason for living'. As I said there is more to life then just living a role. We need to recognize our divinity and ability and live a life, which allows us to love ourselves and the world. It is about our potential and not roles or statistics.

Whether in our lives or when encountering disease we have to ask ourselves, what is my potential? You don't die because of statistics. If you have grown up with love and have self worth you are not afraid to take responsibility and participate in the process of healing your life. If not then you are afraid to participate because the authorities in your life, parents, teachers and clergy have imbued you with the fear of guilt, shame and blame. The by-product of healing your life can be curing your body. I focus on helping people to heal their lives. I learned something from Mother Teresa. She was invited to an anti-war rally and refused to attend. As the people began to leave she said, "But if you ever have a peace rally call me." When we seek to heal our lives we empower ourselves and when we wage a war against cancer or any enemy we empower our enemy.

So work at healing your life and body and eliminating your disease and stop battling and killing because it can have the opposite effect upon you and your body to engage in the battle and worry about being a loser. Death is inevitable but it doesn't mean you lost the battle or failed. Unless you interpret it that way because of the mottoes to die by, and not live by, you heard from your authority figures. I know people who had one of their cats die of lung cancer and they now smoke outdoors because they would rather put up with the inconvenience of smoking outdoors in order to stop killing their cats. Of course they are killing themselves with no conflict of interest or emotions. Nine hundred years ago Maimonides said, "If people took as good care of themselves as they do their animals they would suffer fewer illnesses." So reparent yourself and love yourself and heal your life.

Thoughts and Healing

What we need to do to heal is to turn the curse into a blessing. I ask people to tell me what they're experiencing when I seek to help them. I do not ask only for their diagnosis and what is wrong with them. If they say a wake up call, blessing or new beginning I know they are on the right track, but when they say failure, pressure, draining, confusion, roadblock and more I ask them how those words fit their life. Why? Because when we see what issues are represented by those words and eliminate them from our lives we are healing our lives and helping to cure our bodies. When failure relates to your feeling like a failure as a child because your parents committed suicide then your cancer redirects your life and starts the process of healing.

So I recommend what Nietzsche said, "Love your fate." Which Joseph Campbell explains as accepting that no matter what hell has entered your life to ask yourself, "Why did I need this?" I find when I do this it changes my attitude and the curse becomes a blessing. The darkness of the charcoal becomes a diamond under pressure because it helps me to know myself better and become a more complete human being.

Years ago I was on all the famous talk shows with doctors criticizing me for asking questions about what had happened in people's lives before they became sick and how they can benefit from an illness and more. I was told I was blaming my patients for getting sick. No, I was finding out what had made them vulnerable. Studies now reveal those cancer patients who laugh live longer and that loneliness affects the genes which control immune function. Feeling loved leads you to care for yourself and not be addicted and self-destructive. So you can see why the poet WH Auden would have a doctor, in his poem Miss Gee say, "Cancer's a funny thing. Childless women get it and men when they retire. It's as if there had to be an outlet for their foiled creative fire." My questions were a way to delve into these areas of their lives. Elida Evans, a Jungian, wrote in 1926, in her book *A Psychological Study of Cancer*, that cancer is growth gone wrong and a message to take a new path in your life.

Faith and Healing

I might say the other extreme are the people who have a close relationship with their creator and their faith sustains them, as they know they are of divine origin. I know more than one patient who "went home and left my troubles to God" when they were told there was no hope and no further treatment available and had their so-called incurable cancer disappear. For me it is related to the total peace, which they achieve, like the still pond, because of their faith, hope and love. They surrender and accept and achieve peace and the end of the battle. Records of people who visited Lourdes document this but studies show when you label any water Lourdes Holy Water it also benefits more people.

I also know that religion can cause problems of guilt and some clergy believe that God punishes people with cancer and other diseases or uses cancer to make them more spiritual. My comment is very simple. If you lose your car keys does God want you to walk home? If you said yes, you are living the sermon but if you said no, I would look for my car keys, then when you or other people lose their health help them to find it as you would help them to find their car keys.

Using Imagery and Drawing in Cancer Therapy

I realized how many people were living with guilt, shame and blame due to parents, teachers and clergy when I invited one hundred of my cancer patients to come to a support group so they could live a longer healthier life. I expected many hundreds to show up and less than a dozen women came whom my wife labeled exceptional cancer patients, which became an organization, ECaP. They have been my teachers. I learned from them why people didn't die when they were supposed to and that it was not luck or an error in diagnosis but related to their creating a new life, which they and their body loved.

I began to work with imagery and patient's drawings because of my personal experience doing these things for Dr. Carl Simonton and Dr. Elisabeth Kübler-Ross. I began to see that patients displayed anatomy and knowledge of what was occurring in their bodies through their drawings and dreams. I have yet to meet a physician who has been told during his training that Carl Jung interpreted a dream and correctly diagnosed a brain tumor. It is a vital area that doctors should be informed about and used to help them in a therapeutic way. I used drawings to help me make decisions about whether patients needed surgery or had a medical condition and did not require it.

A simple example, and I show examples when I lecture, was a child with enlarged lymph nodes in her neck. Her mother feared it was a lymphoma, which ran in the family. The child handed me two pictures, one of herself with a swollen neck and the second of a cat with long claws. I told the mother her daughter had Cat Scratch Fever. Her biopsy revealed that to be true.

Mind, Body, Spirit as a Whole

Jung made it very clear that there is a unity within us and mind, body and spirit cannot be separated but are part of our unified whole. We know from the experience of organ transplant recipients, awakening after surgery with memories of the organ donor's life, that memories are stored in our bodies. I know from my experience also that consciousness is non-local and an important part of this healing process. I could write another chapter on the subject but I will simply say that I have gone through, in my life, childhood body memories being recalled during a massage, a near death experience when choking on a toy as a four year old, a past life experience, when asked by a friend over the phone, "Why are you living this life?" and animal communication after having a pet, who had been missing for weeks in Connecticut, be located by an animal intuitive friend who lives in California. Yes, the key is again quieting your mind and communicating with animals or even the dead because I have had that experience and have a mystic friend who has done it for me.

I bring this up because I believe we are all impregnated with the consciousness, which has preceded us, and it affects our life's choices and our health. When we do not become confused and emotionally unhealthy due to this inner knowledge and wisdom but communicate with it we can live our longest and healthiest lives.

I must also say that for me health is not about my body but about my state of mind. I think of Helen Keller as a prime example, as well as quadriplegic mouth painters, victims of thalidomide who have no extremities and more who are healed human beings and living examples for all of us. Perhaps in closing I can quote a veterinarian who learned from the animals she operated upon. Prior to her mastectomy she was an emotional disaster until "I remembered all the animals I operate on amputating legs, jaws and more and they wake up and lick their owner's faces. They know they are here to love and be loved and teach us a few things."

So the ultimate in mind-body healing is to find a role model and to live as if you were the person you want to be expressing your love for the world in your unique way. For those who have difficulty doing this I suggest my role model WWLD, or What Would Lassie Do?

So keep the child in you alive. We are all multiple personalities but those of us who were wounded as children seek to protect their inner personalities from relationships out of fear and that is unhealthy. So learn to love yourself and stop fearing what others think. They are not the problem, you are. Build shrines in your home with mottoes to live by and with your picture, as a child, for you to worship and love.

Be content with what you have
Rejoice in the way things are
And when you realize nothing is lacking
The whole world belongs to you
Lao-Tzu

Part IV

Supplemental Aspects –

Holistic Alternative Treatment

of Lung Cancer

Chapter 7

Nutritional Aspects of Lung Cancer – Kim Dalzell, PhD, RD, LD

Introduction

In my opinion, if you're diagnosed with lung cancer and you receive chemotherapy, radiation or surgery, you are only getting half a cancer treatment plan. Too often, conventional medicine treats the symptoms, and overlooks the cause, of disease.

Researchers have found that poor dietary habits, in addition to tobacco use, are associated with an increased risk of lung cancer. And, those foods and dietary practices that prevent cancer actively fight it or fuel it. So it just makes sense for long-term health to quit smoking and take a serious look at what else you are putting into your mouth. Environmental poisons can trigger the cancer process, but proper nutrition can determine whether or not you get cancer. Food can rebuild cells, stimulate immune system function, protect against chemical and environmental toxins, and promote total body wellness.

Diet and Lung Cancer

How do we know that diet can make a difference when it comes to lung cancer? The rate of smoking is much higher in Japan than in the US, and yet the Japanese (who consume a vegetable-rich diet) have a lower incidence of lung cancer. Their diets offer some protection from the disease.

Both dietary excesses and deficiencies play a role in lung cancer development. Diets low in protein, vitamins A, E, B6, and foliate are associated with reduced immunocompetence. Since protein is found in every cell, it makes sense that a protein deficiency or rapid protein turnover caused by cancer treatment would hinder the immune system. Diets high in saturated fat and refined sugar also suppress immunity. Eating right can help you prevent cancer and restore your body during and after cancer treatment.

Here's how you can take action to beat lung cancer, one step at a time:

Action Steps to Beat Lung Cancer
Step One: Stabilize Your Weight

Many people with lung cancer come into my office with some degree of malnutrition. Newly diagnosed lung cancer patients often have at least one abnormal nutritional parameter (low iron stores, lack of appetite, or rapid weight loss, for example). Why is malnutrition such a threat to your recovery? Cancer causes changes that can alter the level of nutrients your body requires for optimal functioning. Side effects associated with chemotherapy, radiation, and surgery can complicate your ability to eat, absorb, or utilize foods. The final insult comes when a malnourished body can't support treatment goals. When you are poorly nourished, your current treatment may not be as effective, or you might not be able to tolerate further treatments.

Over time, inadequate or improper dietary habits can wreak havoc on the healthiest individuals, even 'healthy' cancer patients. If you don't address dietary deficiencies, cachexia ensues. Think of cachexia as a downward spiral. Every cell in your body requires many nutrients to work effectively. Without the proper fuel, cells can't do their jobs, and debilitation begins. Without an opportunity for rebuilding, the chances of recovery are greatly reduced.

Before you dismiss malnutrition as a condition for the weak and debilitated, understand two things: 1) if you are overweight you are still at risk; and 2) even minor degrees of under nutrition are associated with a marked increased risk of hospital admissions and death. Between 40 and 80% of all cancer patients develop some degree of clinical malnutrition. Don't risk delayed treatment and give cancer a chance to progress while you wait to regain your ability to tolerate treatment!

You can take several steps to make sure your nutritional status is up to par. First of all, address the weakening effects of poor nutrition before they become an issue. Communicate with your doctor. Discuss your risk for malnutrition with your health care providers and let them know you are concerned about your nutritional status. A clinical dietitian should be following your progress throughout your treatment and should be available to discuss your dietary needs or concerns. If you haven't met with a dietitian — ask! A dietitian or nutritionist can help you identify risk factors and devise solutions to any special needs related to your diet.

Although it is better to eat something rather than nothing, what you eat can make a difference in your cancer outcome. If you eat rich, thick ice cream milkshakes and cream soups in an attempt to maintain your weight, you are not providing your body what it needs to heal. With a little planning and some knowledge, you can make better meals that are quick to prepare, taste good, are easy to digest, and support normal cell division and immune function.

One of the easiest ways to add healthy calories to your diet can be achieved by eating good-for-you foods that are calorie dense. Dried fruits like currants and raisins, dates and figs, and dried apples and apricots make great cereal toppers. Eat more bananas, cherries, canned fruit in juice, fruit juice bars, mangoes, pineapple, and plantains. Drink 100% fruit juice with all of your meals. Starchy vegetables such as corn, lima beans, parsnips, peas, potatoes, squash, succotash, and sweet potatoes help you cram in the calories. Eat more calorie-packed cereals such as bran cereals and low-fat granolas. Choose quinoa, whole grain breads and pastas, and wild or brown rice. Add wheat germ to cereals, yogurt, and salads.

Don't load up on whole-fat dairy products. Instead, choose nonfat cheeses and yogurts. Add extra calcium and calories by mixing dry milk powder into foods. Beans brimming with calories include garbanzo, kidney, navy, and pinto. Eat more bluefish, chub, herring, mackerel, salmon, sardines, swordfish, and tuna, which contain healthy fats. Try lite soymilk, tempeh, textured vegetable protein, and lite tofu. Add extra virgin olive or canola oil to beans, greens, pasta, potatoes, chicken, or fish. Choose tuna packed in oil. Top salads or sandwiches with slices of avocado.

Testing for Malnutrition

On the clinical front, blood analysis can be helpful to risk of malnutrition. Very commonly, blood is drawn to determine serum albumin levels, which are considered a fairly reliable indicator of protein status, especially when looking at malnutrition in later stages. Serum prealbumin can be used to determine earlier stage protein deficiencies, but most doctors do not routinely order this lab test. Ask whether this test would help the doctor assess your overall health status.

Albumin is a carrier protein that is also responsible for maintaining normal distribution of water within the body. If you notice edema (water retention) around your abdomen or extremities, you may not be getting adequate calories or protein in your diet. Serum albumin levels lower than 3.5 mg/dl are correlated with an increased risk of malnutrition. What can you do if your albumin is low? First, follow up with your health care professional to create a plan of action to stabilize this component. Your nutritionist may have you evaluate your diet for calorie and protein adequacy. Often, a high-calorie high-protein supplemental drink mix is suggested when the albumin drops below this level. Prescription appetite stimulants may be in order as well, so ask your doctor about which medications can help to rev up your desire to eat.

Advanced Nutritional Support

If high-calorie shakes, appetite stimulants, and other dietary modifications don't help you maintain your weight, you may need advanced nutritional support. Advanced nutritional support used as a complementary therapy to basic cancer treatment can decrease the risk of further deterioration, improve some nutritional and immunological parameters, avoid health complications associated with malnutrition, and enhance quality of life. Nutritional support techniques used in cancer patients have reduced complication rates of surgery by 33%! Additionally, survival rates improved, without affecting tumor growth. Take note of this fact: some doctors avoid using advanced nutritional support fearing that they will feed the cancer. Today, we know that just isn't so! Your nutritionist and doctor can assess your need for advanced nutritional support. Advanced nutritional support can be delivered into your gastrointestinal tract (enteral feeding) or blood vessels (parenteral feeding).

Enteral feedings, commonly called tube feedings, are best suited for people who can still eat, digest, and assimilate foods through their gastrointestinal tract. A tube is placed surgically or by an endoscope in an outpatient procedure. This form of advanced nutritional support is the most cost-effective and best for optimal delivery of nutrients to your body. The rule of thumb is, if the gut works, use it. So, if your gastrointestinal tract is functioning, this method of nutritional support is appropriate for you.

Intravenous feeding, often called total parenteral nutrition (TPN), is reserved for individuals who are unable to assimilate nutrients through the gastrointestinal tract. Nutrients in a liquid solution are infused intravenously. Total parenteral nutrition requires a surgeon to place a catheter into either a peripheral vein (for short-term feedings) or a central vein such as the subclavian or internal jugular vein (for long-term feedings).

As with any surgical procedure, there is an increased risk of infection, so care must be taken to keep the catheter site clean. As with enteral nutritional therapies, there are different routes and methods of administration, formulas, and complications associated with TPN. Your surgeon and nurse will review all of this information with you prior to your discharge from the hospital. Total parenteral nutrition can be administered at home, and home health agencies provide appropriate follow-up care. TPN and home health care for TPN are covered by most health insurance policies.

Step Two: Lose Weight If You Need To

Several years ago, a study published in the *American Journal of Epidemiology* revealed that being overweight is tied to lung cancer risk. This study was the first to link obesity with lung cancer. What's the connection between fat and lung cancer? Turns out, excessive weight may elevate serum levels of insulin-like growth factor (IGF-1), which can cause cancer cells to grow and spread. Other studies also suggest that higher levels of cancer-causing chemicals might be stored in excess fat tissue or that extra calories provide fuel for increased cell proliferation.

The American Institute for Cancer Research recommends limiting weight gain to eleven pounds during adulthood. Most of us exceed this recommendation as we age. Often, changing what you eat can prompt weight loss and this jump-start to a leaner figure can be a strong motivational factor for continued adherence to a more healthful diet. Don't forget the other part of the weight maintenance equation: Physical activity can help increase muscle mass and burn calories. Discuss with your medical doctor which forms of physical activity may be right for you.

As you adjust to new eating and activity habits, your new energy requirements will be established as your body composition changes. Talk with a registered dietitian who can help you design a meal plan for realistic and safe weight loss. Avoid strict or fad diets in an attempt to lose weight because quick weight loss strips the body of lean muscle tissue, deprives the body of valuable nutrients needed for growth and repair, and can reduce the fighting capacity of your immune system. If you need to lose weight, strive for a weight trim of about 1–2 pounds per week

Step Three: Maintain a Healthy Gut

Do you ever wonder what happens to that 12-ounce porterhouse steak after you've eaten it? Let's take a walk down the digestive tract and find out. The process of digestion begins with the sight and smell of food. In fact, the brain signals enzymes in your mouth to be released just at the thought of food. After the food is chewed, mixed with saliva, and swallowed, it travels down the esophagus, a long pipe extending from the throat to the top of the stomach. The stomach is the key to the whole digestive process, releasing hydrochloric acid to break apart proteins. The stomach muscles contract to churn the food into a mixture called chyme.

Digestive enzymes secreted from the pancreas work on the partially digested food particles to prepare them for absorption in the small intestine.

About 90% of all nutrients are absorbed by the intestines and distributed to cells throughout your body. Fluid and a few other nutrients are absorbed in the colon. Whatever the body doesn't use is eliminated through the colon, and any waste is expelled out of the rectum. Digestion is much more complicated than this, but even with this brief overview, it is easy to see that many steps are required for food to be formulated into body fuel. This is why it is so important to make sure your digestion is on track

There are many opportunities for cancer treatment, or the cancer itself, to affect the intricate functioning of the GI tract. Chemotherapy and radiation have the potential to interrupt the delicate chemical and physical mechanisms needed for the digestion and absorption of food. Because the gastrointestinal tract has rapid cellular turnover, it can be affected by cell-destroying treatments more severely than other parts of the body. Diarrhea, constipation, excessive bloating and cramping, and other uncomfortable and potentially serious side effects can be very challenging obstacles to health.

The risk of malnutrition is increased, especially in cancers of the head or neck or GI tract. Chewing or swallowing problems occur with treatment involving the surgical removal or chemical destruction of the tongue, neck muscles, salivary glands, or tooth structures. Radiation to the chest can adversely affect the function of the esophagus and increase incidence of reflux and achalasia, which is a lack of enzyme activity. Early satiety due to physical blockage caused by tumor invasion into the GI tract wall can also be a problem. Strictures, which are involuntary closures of the esophagus, make swallowing or food passing into the stomach impossible.

If your gastrointestinal tract does not work very well, you won't be able to utilize all the nutrients you consume. To achieve a balance of beneficial bacteria in the intestines, eat yogurt or take a probiotic supplement on a regular basis. I often see lung cancer patients who have problems with early satiety – they fill up easily and can't eat very much at one sitting.

Eating small, frequent meals and taking digestive enzymes can aid in the absorption of nutrients to support healthy cells. Digestive enzymes have also been shown to have anticancer action because they have the capability of breaking down the tissue that covers encapsulated tumors and decreasing the 'spreadability' of cancer cells. Bromelain, an enzyme found in pineapple, has demonstrated antimetastatic properties in laboratory animals with implanted lung cancer cells.

Constipation can be a serious problem for individuals with lung cancer. Infrequent bowel movements increase the risk of toxic buildup that can contribute to poor overall health. Effective elimination clears harmful bile acids, dilutes carcinogens, and promotes the growth of beneficial gut bacteria. Optimal bowel transit time (the amount of time it takes food to enter through the mouth, go through the digestive tract and exit out through the stool) is twelve to eighteen hours. If you have hard stools, difficulty defecating, or do not have a bowel movement at least twice a day, you are constipated. The main cause for constipation is poor fluid intake. Other causes for constipation include dietary intake, recent bowel surgery, and laxative abuse. Chemotherapies that may cause constipation include Navelbine and Temodal.

To combat constipation, eat a high-fiber diet, which promotes bowel regularity. Supplemental powders containing oat bran, rice bran, and psyllium attract water into feces, bulking up the stool for easy passage. Avoid milk and milk products if you are lactose intolerant. Lactose intolerance can cause constipation.

Limit caffeine-containing beverages such as coffee, tea, and cocoa or chocolate products. Caffeine tends to pull water out of the colon. Limit binding foods such as bananas, apples, and rice. Drink at least 64 oz of purified water per day. Stimulate bowel movements by drinking warm liquids, such as broth or herbal tea, prior to meals.

Natural laxatives include prunes, prune juice, and ground flaxseeds. Sienna and cascara sagrada are cathartic herbs, but may be very powerful for weakened individuals, so use with caution. Limit the use of laxatives, as bowels can become lazy with regular use. Avoid mineral oil, which interferes with the absorption of calcium and fat-soluble vitamins. Explore medication alternatives to pain relievers, antidepressants, or antacids containing aluminum, which are constipating.

Finally, see a gastroenterologist to rule out an intestinal blockage if you have small, ribbon-like stools. Bowel obstructions will usually cause severe cramping and vomiting. If left untreated, the distended bowel can rupture.

The flipside of constipation is diarrhea. When you have diarrhea, food is whisked through your GI tract so quickly that it can't be adequately absorbed and assimilated into cells. This rapid transit of nutrients leads to weight loss, dehydration, immune system depression, physical weakness, and malnutrition.

Various chemotherapy drugs can cause diarrhea. Navelbine, Taxotere, Taxol, and 5-FU can have toxic effects on the intestinal lining of the bowels. Many digestive disorders, such as lactose intolerance, inflammatory bowel disease, and irritable bowel syndrome can also lead to diarrhea. Get your bowels in order by completely chewing your food to aid digestion. Enzymes in the digestive tract can readily break down the smaller food components of well-chewed food, ensuring optimal absorption into the intestinal wall. Eat a high-fiber diet or try the BRAT diet. The BRAT diet can be used for a few days to help control severe diarrhea. This diet is named for the selection of foods that bind: bananas, rice, apples, and toast.

Rehydrate with fruit and veggie juices (naturally high in potassium). Prolonged loss of fluids can lead to dehydration and mineral imbalance.

Add soy protein or carob powders to drink mixtures. Soy powder has been used to reduce diarrhea induced by chemotherapy. Stimulate digestive enzyme activity with pungent foods such as garlic, ginger, curry, and onions. Raw foods, which contain live digestive enzymes, contribute to digestion as well. Avoid foods or drinks that stimulate loose bowels such as prunes, other dried fruits, prune juice, sugary sports drinks such as Gatorade, juices with added sugar, and so on. Avoid sugarless candies and gums that contain sugar alcohols such as mannitol, xylitol, or sorbitol. Even small amounts of these products can cause diarrhea. Hot foods stimulate peristalsis so you may want to eat more cold or room temperature foods. Raw beans, broccoli, cauliflower, brussels sprouts, and cabbage may be difficult to digest.

Avoid all dairy products except for yogurt if you are lactose intolerant. Digestive enzymes can help with possible pancreatic digestive insufficiency. Probiotics that contain live cells can improve gastrointestinal function. Look for acidophilus supplements that contain *Saccharomyces bouldardii,* yeast that has been used to treat diarrhea induced by antibiotics.

Herbs used to treat parasite-induced diarrhea include goldenseal, Oregon grape, and grapefruit seed extract. Zinc and B12 may be needed to replace losses due to excessive diarrhea. See a gastroenterologist to determine whether you have parasites or bacterial overgrowth. Your doctor will determine if you need an antidiarrheal medication such as Kaopectate or Lomotil to slow bowel movements or thicken stools. Kaopectate has no side effects, but Lomotil can cause bloating and nausea.

Swallowing difficulties can occur with low levels of saliva, which may be caused by surgery to the salivary glands or neck region, radiation to the head, neck and chest area, or chemotherapies that cause transitional dryness of the mouth.

Here are some easy things you can do to help with swallowing challenges. Stimulate saliva by sucking on lemon drops, root beer barrels, peppermint hard candy, frozen fruit juices or ice chips. Add citrus wedges to your purified water. Take over-the-counter saliva replacements such as Oral Balance mouth moisturizing gel. Fill a spray bottle with water and spray liquid into your mouth periodically throughout the day. Add fat-free broths to rice, potatoes, pastas, and breads. Consume more broth-based soups as meals. Avoid dry or salty foods, which tend to increase the need for fluid. Try recipes that incorporate sweet pickles, soy sauce, and other aromatic foods to stimulate the appetite and get your mouth watering.

Visit your dentist more often; saliva is responsible for washing away bacteria from teeth surfaces. Biotene toothpaste, gum, and mouthwash is available over the counter for dry mouth and maintenance of healthy oral flora.

Taste changes can be a serious problem for individuals with lung cancer. Changes occur with chemotherapy because taste buds are rapidly destroyed. Other situations that can alter taste sensations include radiation to the neck or chest region, bacterial overgrowth of candida, mouth surgery, and nutritional deficiencies. Avoid red meat, which may taste like metal. Instead, choose mild tasting fish, soy products, and lean chicken and turkey as protein sources.

As a daily minimum, you should consume at least three servings of fruit and five servings of vegetables each day. Keep in mind that this goal is appropriate for someone who requires about 1,500 calories per day. As caloric requirements increase, so should fruit and vegetable intake. For example, if you need 2,000 calories per day, you should shoot for an intake goal of eight to ten servings of produce each day. That may seem like a lot, but for fighting cancer, more produce is better.

Researchers at Johns Hopkins Medical Institute found greater levels of antioxidants in individuals who consumed eight to ten servings of fruits and vegetables each day as compared to individuals who ate fewer servings. These antioxidants offer protection against cell damage and support tissue healing. Numerous studies have reported a positive association between consuming produce and preventing lung cancer. Nature has packed cancer-fighting phytochemicals into almost every kind of fruit and vegetable.

Maximize the health potential of your fruits and vegetables by eating vegetables and fruits that have deep, rich colors. The darker a plant is, the greater the phytochemical potential. Sweet potatoes are better than white potatoes.

One serving of romaine lettuce contains almost eight times as much vitamin A as a serving of iceberg lettuce. Get the picture?

Eat a variety of fruits and vegetables each day. Don't limit your vegetable choices to only broccoli and cabbage. While both of these vegetables have outstanding nutritional profiles, they can contribute only a fraction of the important cancer-fighting chemicals to your diet.

Consuming a mixed bag of plants gives you a well-rounded dose of a variety of phytochemicals and provides an opportunity for the chemicals to work together in a more powerful way. Be sure to eat whole natural fruits and vegetables. Consume phyto-chemical-rich plants in their raw or slightly cooked form. Eating uncooked, unprocessed plants contributes enzymes for digestion and provides the highest levels of nutrients. Lightly steamed vegetables retain some of the nutrients lost with other cooking methods. If you can't eat fresh produce, frozen produce is your next best choice. Use canned fruits or vegetables as a last resort. Canned produce has been stripped of fiber-rich peelings, has fewer nutrients, and may contain added sweeteners or sodium. The best tip I can offer you is to ask yourself at every meal, "Where are my fruits and veggies?" Make sure you can see the answer on your plate.

The National Cancer Institute offers these serving size guide-lines for fruits and vegetables:

1 medium fruit or 1/2 cup of small or diced fruit
1/2 cup 100% juice
1/4 cup dried fruit
1/2 cup raw non-leafy or cooked vegetables
1 cup raw leafy vegetables
1/2 cup cooked beans or peas

As you can see, a serving of fruit or vegetables is reasonable in size but I have rarely met someone, including myself, who can consume this many servings of produce per day. While all produce is powerful, there are some specific plants that have been identified specifically for their anti-lung cancer activity, so be sure to focus your diet on foods that contain these compounds: Anthocyanidins are powerful water-soluble antioxidants that have been found to support cardiovascular function and protect against macular degeneration and cataracts. Antitumor effects using anthocyanidin extracts have been demonstrated on lung cancer cells.

Grape seed proanthocyanidin extract has shown cytotoxic activity towards human lung, breast and stomach cancer cells. Find anthocyanidins in bilberry, blackberries, cherries, cranberries, currants, eggplant, lentils, plums, raspberries, red cabbage, red grapes, red wine, rhubarb, and strawberries.

Beta-carotene, which can be converted to vitamin A in the body, is one of six hundred identified carotenoids. Diets high in beta-carotene provide immune protection and antioxidant benefit. Research has demonstrated that beta-carotene offers protection against cervical and lung cancers and helps to modulate human prostate cancer cell growth. Caution: dietary sources of beta-carotene are safe to consume; dietary supplements containing isolated beta-carotene are not. Further explanation of this rule will be detailed in the last step on supplementation.

Other carotenoids such as alpha carotene, cryptoxanthin, lutein, lycopene, and zeaxanthin also contribute to disease prevention, a point that helps support the benefit of whole foods rather than isolated nutrient supplementation. Several studies have shown that both single and multiple carotenes prevent carcinogens from entering cells and help repair genetic injury. By this action carotenes may play a protective role against tumor progression associated with oxidative damage.

Food sources include arugula, broccoli, butternut squash, cantaloupe, carrots, chard, collard greens, daikon, endive, horseradish, kale, mango, mustard greens, Napa cabbage, nectarines, oranges, papaya, peach, peppers, pumpkin, sorrel, spinach, star fruit, tangerine, tomato, turnip greens, and yams.

Catechins, or tannins, are chemically active compounds that have been linked to lower rates of gastrointestinal and lung cancer. These flavanols are seven times more potent than vitamin E as an antioxidant. They inhibit the activation of carcinogens and have demonstrated anti-inflammatory, probiotic, and antimicrobial properties in human, animal, and test tube studies.

Researchers analyzed the diets of nearly 600 people in Hawaii who had lung cancer and compared them with diets in a matched group without cancer. They found that people who ate the most apples, white grapefruit and onions – food especially high in the flavonoid quercetin – were almost 50% less likely to develop lung cancer. Other food sources of flavonoids include apple juice, berries, black tea, grapes, green tea, peaches, persimmons, plums, red wine, and strawberries.

Ellagic acid, a flavonoid known to act as a free radical scavenger, may prevent mutation of genes. It is a proven cancer fighter, stopping tumor growth in esophageal and lung cancer animal studies. Food sources include apples, blackberries, cranberries, grapes, raspberries, strawberries, and walnuts.

Phenolic compounds such as chlorogenic, caffeic, and ferulic acids block the formation of nitrosamines. These cancer-causing agents are formed when the stomach acid converts dietary nitrates (from bacon, ham, hot dogs and other processed meats) into nitrosamines. We see a direct connection between nitro amine formation and lung cancer. Caffeic acid is an anti-inflammatory agent that has been shown to increase cancer cell death. Food sources include broccoli, cabbage, carrots, cherries, citrus fruit, eggplant, grapefruit, oranges, parsley, pears, peppers, prunes, and tomato. Phytoestrogens such as daidzein and genistein are found in soybeans. They have the most active blocking potential against estrogen receptors in the breast and ovaries. Lignans, coumestans, and saponins are weaker phytoestrogens. Consumption of these plant hormones has been linked to a decreased risk of many cancers including lung cancer.

Research has shown that both daidzein and genistein enhance the activation of human natural killer cells. A recent study has demonstrated the significant antimutagenic activity of saponins. Food sources include bean sprouts, broccoli, cabbage, cucumbers, eggplant, flaxseeds, peppers, soymilk, soybeans, squash, tofu, and whole grains.

In terms of fighting lung cancer, eating more fruits and vegetables is top priority! It does take effort, but with all the proven benefits of plants for controlling cancer, it is an important thing to do. Develop a routine of eating fruits and vegetables at every meal. Once you get into the habit of eating plants, you'll definitely miss them when you don't eat them. Look at the following list of suggestions for adding more fruits and vegetables to your diet. Then come up with some of your own strategies to meet your goal of 9–13 servings each day!

Add grated zucchini and carrots to ground turkey, beef, or textured vegetable protein. Shape into burgers or loaf form and grill or bake.

Dice up colorful peppers and onions and add them to potato wedges. Toss olive oil, chopped garlic cloves, and a quarter teaspoon of thyme. Roast in an oven for about thirty minutes or until the potatoes are tender.

Replace half the meat in lasagna or spaghetti sauces with sliced or grated vegetables.

Carry a bag of petite carrots with you to work. Add to a sandwich in place of fries, chips, or potato or macaroni salad.

Top fish with a citrus chutney or hearty salsa. Add zip to your chicken by adding a cherry sauce; bake cinnamon sprinkled apple wedges with pork chops.

Dress up homemade or commercial soups by adding canned or frozen vegetables. Just like that, you've added a half serving of vegetables per one cup of soup!

I think it's important to say a few words about juicing. While juicing a cup or so per day may be an answer to obtaining more fruits and veggies for some of you, I typically do not recommend getting the majority of your produce in a liquid form. Lots of juice fills you up quickly, doesn't typically provide enough fiber, and may negatively impact your immune system by elevating blood sugar levels. Maintaining a normalized blood sugar level is very important to fighting cancer cell growth.

In twenty years of helping cancer patients, the dilemma of how to obtain consistently large amounts of quality produce, safe from pesticides and herbicides, on a daily basis is one of the most challenging aspects to solid nutritional therapy. I believe it is necessary for every cancer patient – for that matter, for everyone – to supplement with a whole food product.

Based on the large body of research, including a study being conducted at MD Anderson Cancer Center and a clinical trial of cancer patients funded by the National Institutes of Health, I use and recommend Juice Plus+. This is the only whole food supplement I have found that is backed up by numerous, double-blind, placebo controlled human studies. I highly recommend you take this, along with a goal to eat more fruits and veggies. You can review the research on Juice Plus+ at my patient information site: www.juiceplusmed.com.

Step Four: Cut the Fat

Dietary fat can alter inflammatory conditions, immune system function, and impact lung cancer. Eating high-fat foods, especially those containing saturated fats and polyunsaturated fats, appears to be linked to lung cancer risk. Diets high in eggs and other cholesterol-rich foods possibly increase the risk of lung cancer. This doesn't mean you should avoid eggs entirely, but they should not be consumed daily.

One of the fastest ways to remove the bad fat from your diet is to take a quick look at your pantry shelves. Do you see any products that contain hydrogenated fats? Look closely at any packaged convenience foods such as rice or pasta mixes, crackers, and ready-to-eat cereals. Do they list trans fats on the label? Perhaps in the ingredients section you see the words 'hydrogenated' or 'partially hydrogenated'? If so, throw these foods away!

Next, take out the dinners, pizza, and packets of seasoned vegetables from the freezer. See any dangerous fats there? Open up your refrigerator door. Look at your dairy products, processed cheeses, coffee creamer, and margarine. Every food product you buy that contains hydrogenated or partially hydrogenated oils has health-damaging potential.

Butter is better than margarine for several reasons. Butter, because of its fatty acid content, is perfect for high-heat cooking methods. Margarine is not suitable for frying or sautéing. Butter does contain some naturally occurring trans-fatty acids, but the hydrogenation process used to make margarine creates substantially more trans-fatty acids. Margarine is also a source of undesirable aluminum and nickel. If you are worried about environmental contaminants, you can avoid pesticide and hormones by purchasing organic butter.

If there is one type of fat we tend to be 'deficient' in, it would be the super unsaturated omega-3 fatty acids. At least 15% of your daily calories (60% of your total fat allowance) should come from fats that contain monounsaturated and omega-3 fatty acids. These omega-3 superunsaturates can slow tumor growth in lung cancer, decrease the metastatic properties of cancer cells, and increase cancer patient survival time.

Extra virgin olive oil is the top choice for monounsaturated fatty acids. Unrefined, essential fatty acids are found in cold water fish, flaxseeds, and in lesser amounts, soybeans and walnuts. The oil should be stored in a dark, opaque container and the label should state 'extra virgin' to ensure that the oil has not been refined. Be sure to buy cold-pressed oil. This processing technique eliminates heat destruction of the seed or oil. For intense flavor and the most phytochemicals, choose the deeper golden-green oils.

You should eat at least one meal of fish per week. Eating fish will provide you with an excellent source of protein and will help you reduce your total saturated fat intake. Most of the essential oils are found under the skin, so cold water fish are best eaten with their skins on. What kinds of fish should you be fishing for? Atlantic salmon, sardines, and farmed Coho salmon and rainbow trout have between two and four omega-3 fat grams per serving. Other fish such as mackerel, flounder, halibut, and canned tuna contain less than one omega-3 fat gram per serving.

Even if you consume fish more than once a week, you should supplement your diet with omega-3 fatty acids in order to obtain therapeutic levels of these essential oils. Simply add omega-3 fatty acid oil or supplements to your nutritional regimen. This is an appealing option for those who would rather take a pill than eat fish every day. I recommend a therapeutic grade fish oil. A couple of brands that have been tested for impurities include Nordic Naturals and Carlson. Flaxseeds contain more omega-3 fatty acids than fish oil, but the acids in flax have to be converted in the body to EPA (the substance found in fish oil that exhibits beneficial health properties). With adequate levels of B3, B6, vitamin C, magnesium, and zinc, your body easily makes this conversion. One to two tablespoons of flax per day is a typical dosage recommendation. Flaxseeds have many health benefits. They are rich in minerals such as potassium and magnesium, and in vitamins such as niacin, riboflavin, C and E, and carotenes. Mucilage, a water-soluble fiber found in flax, aids constipation, moderates blood sugar levels, and soothes digestive disorders. One ounce of flaxseed meal contains a whopping eleven grams of dietary fiber. Barlean's has ground-up flax that can be sprinkled over cereal, blended into muffins or breads, and mixed into health shakes.

Step Five: Eat Soy

Consume an average of two servings of soy foods daily. Soy, which doesn't contain saturated fat, is a high-protein alternative to animal foods that has slowed tumor growth and limited the metastatic properties of various cancer cells. Researchers found that the soy isoflavone called genistein was able to induce lung cancer cell death.

Isoflavones, along with protein, vitamin E, omega-3 fatty acids, saponins, phytosterols, phytates, fiber, and oligosaccharides, appear to work together to contribute to overall health in a number of ways, including reduction of menopausal symptoms, possibly decreasing risk of heart disease, regulation of blood sugar levels, support of bone health, and a good choice for individuals who are lactose intolerant and can't consume dairy products.

Soybeans are extremely versatile and have been made into a variety of foods. Soybeans by themselves have a very mild flavor and should be combined with other ingredients to help create a flavorful product.

Most soy foods vary in protein and fat content. Tofu and soymilk, for example, come in regular and lite (reduced fat) versions. Texturized vegetable protein and soy protein isolates, unlike other soy products, contain very little fat. Most soymilks contain about seven grams of protein per serving, but this can vary depending on the brand you buy. Flavored soymilk and silken tofu typically contain less protein, so make sure you read the labels to choose the best product for your needs.

Whole soybeans are available in health food stores and supermarkets in bags or bulk bins. Dry soybeans expand two to three times when cooked in liquid; they should be soaked to decrease cooking time and enhance the digestibility of the beans. Edamame, green soybeans, are picked before they reach maturity and look like green peas. Soybeans are eaten as a side dish or used in salads and soups. Roasted soybeans, called soy nuts, are a crunchy snack. Read labels carefully to make sure hydrogenated oils were not used in the roasting process.

Soymilk is a nutty flavored liquid extracted from soybeans. Soymilk comes in a variety of flavors such as chocolate, vanilla, carob, almond, and plain. Read product labels carefully because the protein content varies in different brands of soymilk. Choose lite soymilks because they are lower in fat. You can drink soymilk straight from the carton, pour it over cold cereal, or use it for cooking or baking. West Soy and Eden Soy are top brands to look for. Tofu, or soybean curd, is made by curdling fresh, hot soymilk. The curds are generally pressed together to form a solid block. Consistency varies by type. Firm tofu is dense and retains its shape well. It is used in stir-fry recipes, soups, or on the grill. Soft tofu is less dense and used in Oriental soups or in recipes that call for blended tofu. Silken tofu is creamy like custard. It is often pureed or blended and used to make salad dressings, dips, pasta sauces, desserts, and smoothies.

Tempeh, pronounced 'tem-pay', is a cultured soy food made with soybeans and grain. It has a dense, chewy texture and can be added to sandwiches, soup, and casseroles, or it can be grilled and served next to rice. If you don't like tofu because it lacks texture, you might like tempeh.

Texturized soy protein is made from compressed soy flour. It comes in granular, flake, or chunk form, and in a variety of flavors. When it is rehydrated with boiling water, texturized soy protein has a grainy texture similar to meat. It is found in commercial products as a meat extender or is pressed into patties to form veggie burgers. Read labels carefully. Some veggie burgers are a combination of grains and vegetables and do not contain soy at all.

There are a few circumstances where I do not recommend a large intake of soy foods. Women with a personal medical history of estrogen-dependent cancers (breast, ovarian, uterine or other gynecological cancers) should consume soy sparingly. More studies are needed to determine whether soy ingestion is safe for any estrogen-dependent cancers.

The American Dietetic Association suggests that to play it safe, women with breast cancer or women using Tamoxifen should completely avoid dietary soy supplements. While soy protein powders or pills contain high doses of genistein and daidzein, food sources of soy contain less concentrated levels of isoflavones and offer a variety of health benefits.

For these reasons, health care professionals suggest soy foods may be safely consumed in moderation (two to three servings per week) by women with estrogen-sensitive tumors. Just to make sure there is no confusion: for individuals with lung cancer, soy intake on a daily basis is recommended. I like the whole food approach, so eating soy foods is safer and better than consuming isolated soy pills or powders.

Step Six: Cut the Sweets

Have you ever heard that sugar feeds cancer? We all know that simple sugars, the sweetener most often found in desserts, candies, and soft drinks, are detrimental to health. Diets high in sugar have been linked to a number of health problems, including diabetes, hypoglycemia, chronic constipation, intestinal gas, asthma, candida infections, headaches, obesity, inflammatory bowel disease, and tooth decay. Eating sugar affects cancer as well. Researchers have been able to link processed, refined starches and sugars to cancer development in three ways:

It elevates insulin levels.
It creates a toxic burden.
It negatively impacts immunity.

Tumors, just like normal cells, prefer carbohydrates as their main source of energy. When you eat sweets your blood sugar rises rapidly. In response to all this sugar in your blood, the insulin hormone is released by the pancreas. Insulin helps cells to use the sugar as energy and brings blood sugar levels back to normal. When you eat too much sugar, a large amount of insulin is produced and circulates in the blood. High insulin levels cause precancerous cells to gobble up sugar, accelerating their growth into fully formed cancer cells.

Eating sugary foods, which have a tendency to be low in fiber, slows the movement of the GI tract and contributes to constipation. High-sugar diets also increase production of secondary bile acids. These carcinogenic compounds contribute to a toxic GI environment and have been linked to cancer.

Nourishing the cells that protect you from foreign invaders is a number one priority. A constant threat of viral or bacterial infection, in conjunction with destructive cancer treatments, increases immune system vulnerability. Add a high-sugar diet to the equation and you short circuit your immunity. Elevated insulin levels slow the release of growth hormones, which in turn reduce white blood cell production.

Limit refined sugar and flour intake to less than 10% of your total calories. Sugar, as well as other highly processed carbohydrates, can raise blood sugar levels, creating an environment favorable for cancer cell growth and suppressed immunity. Your blood sugar response to certain foods is very unique. Your own physiology has a lot to do with how quickly a food is digested and then released into your bloodstream. To balance blood sugar levels, avoid foods that trigger blood sugar peaks. Limit sugary confections, desserts, and other sweet treats.

Be sure to eat high-fiber foods. Diets rich in fiber create a slow, even energy uptake. Choose whole grain breads, buckwheat pasta, and brown rice in place of white bread, pasta, and rice products. Combine high-sugar foods with protein. The release of sugar into the bloodstream is slowed down when meat, eggs, or other protein sources accompany potatoes, fruit, or other carbohydrates. Don't eat fruit or drink fruit juice alone; combine with nuts or seeds. Finally, if you have dessert, eat it at the end of a protein-based meal.

Hidden sugars are everywhere, so be on the look out! Sugar goes by a number of names, so inspect the ingredient section of food labels for the following terms: sugar, sucrose, dextrose, fructose, powdered sugar, maple sugar, brown sugar, corn syrup, levulose, high fructose corn syrup, honey, milk sugar, lactose, and maltose.

Soft drinks, flavored beverages, and fruit drinks are loaded with sugar. Did you know that one can of soda contains between 7 and 10 teaspoons of sugar? Most colorful sports drinks used to replace sodium and potassium after strenuous workouts contain tons of sugar. The only time to drink a sports drink is when you are dehydrated from severe diarrhea or vomiting. Check the label on flavored bottled waters. Usually, they contain a sweetener as a flavor enhancer.

Canned fruits come packed in heavy, light, and fruit-juice based syrups. Make sure you take a good long look at the label and purchase the fruit that is packed in juice or light syrup. Choosing 'lite' fruits will reduce your intake of sugar by at least 50%.

Low-fat bakery products such as crackers, cookies, and cakes are often high in sugar because while there is less fat in these products, the fat has been replaced with sugar. Consider preparing baked goods from scratch to control the amount of sugar in them. Children's cereals are very high in sugar, but adults' cereals can be too. A peek at the labels of some granolas and oat bran cereals will convince you of this.

It's important to mention something about sugar substitutes. Sugar substitutes are found most often in drinks, baked goods, yogurts, puddings, and frozen desserts. Some people use sugar substitutes to help them lose weight. While it is true that most sugar substitutes don't provide significant calories, research has proven they do not contribute to long-term weight loss. Animal studies have shown that saccharin (found in Sweet'N Low for example) is a tumor promoter in the bladder, lungs, and other organs. Aspartame (found in NutraSweet and Equal) has been linked to neurological disorders. Sucralose, also called Splenda, is the newest approved low-calorie sweetener to grace our consumer market. It's about six hundred times sweeter than sugar, is made from sugar, and is calorie free. Safety studies suggest this is a nontoxic product, but I believe that an herbal alternative sweetener called stevia may be a better choice than artificial sweeteners. Stevia contains no calories and has been shown to lower blood sugar levels. Stevia's flavor is quite acceptable, although some patients have reported that it has a mild licorice aftertaste. Stevia comes in powder and liquid form.

Step Seven: Drink Right

A nationwide food consumption survey found that chronic mild dehydration was commonplace among Americans. To be well hydrated and flush your system of toxins, you should consume at least twelve cups of fluid per day if you are a man, nine cups of fluid per day if you are a woman. Drinking adequate fluid flushes toxins out of the body and allows for optimal nutrient movement in and out of the cells and tissues. I recommend drinking reverse osmosis treated or distilled water. Some studies show drinking green and black tea offers a protective effect against lung cancer.

Studies indicate that the risk of developing lung cancer increased incrementally as daily alcohol intake increases. I suggest you limit alcohol consumption to special occasions or avoid alcohol entirely.

Step Eight: Detoxify Your Diet, One Step at a Time

Your body normally has the capacity to dispose of harmful substances and can miraculously inactivate, remove, or change toxic substances in an attempt to prevent a buildup of waste products. The organs primarily responsible for detoxification include the gastrointestinal tract, kidney, and liver. The lymphatic system and skin also have specific elimination functions. At the cellular level, compounds such as superoxide dismutase (SOD) and glutathione peroxidase act as free radical scavengers and assist in the excretion of potential cancer-causing agents.

With all of these cleansing mechanisms in place, how can toxicity occur? If you have constipation or your immune system is compromised, wastes tend to build up in the body, leak through the intestinal wall, and flow into the liver. The liver is primarily responsible for clearing the body of poisons. If the liver is overtaxed, toxins simply circulate in the blood, taking shelter in the brain, nervous system, and fatty tissues. Healthy cells are injured when exposed to these toxins. Studies have shown that individuals with compromised detoxification systems are the most susceptible to developing a chronic disease such as cancer.

Think about your ability to detoxify. How will you combat the pesticides, hormones, and antibiotics that saturate our food supply? How will your body purge itself of the effects of radiation, chemotherapy, and any prescription drugs that you might have used to diminish treatment side effects? If you smoke, stop now. Continuing to smoke can reduce the benefit of natural therapies and increase your risk for other diseases.

It has been estimated that up to 90% of all cancers can be linked to the environment, with diet being the number one contributing factor. When you eat foods that are unadulterated, you help your body clear unwanted pollutants so it can begin healing. A detoxification program isn't going to help much if you aren't making appropriate dietary choices to begin with.

Detoxifying your diet doesn't have to be overwhelming. Start slowly and make adjustments one step at a time. Begin by reducing your intake of sugar, caffeine, and alcohol. Move toward a chemical-free diet by refraining from artificial sweet-eners, colors, and flavoring agents. Unadulterated foods leave little for the liver to clear out.

Read food package labels to identify and dismiss any foods that contain sulfites, nitrates, and phosphates. These additives are linked to a number of health problems. Avoid foods made with hydrogenated and partially hydrogenated fats and chemically extracted oils. Processed fats are toxic to our cells, and rancid fats increase the free radicals in the body. Limit high temperature cooking (grilling or broiling) of meats, which contribute to the formation of potentially cancer-causing chemicals called heterocyclic amines.

Buy organically grown, hormone- and antibiotic-free products. Steer clear of foods that have been genetically engineered or irradiated. Consume a plant-based diet. Eat more whole grains, seeds, nuts, and legumes. Fiber is essential for healthy gut function, aids in reducing blood glucose and cholesterol levels, and helps to detoxify the body by binding to carcinogenic materials in the colon. Eat at least five to nine servings of antioxidant-rich fruits and vegetables every day. Bright yellow and deep orange produce contains immune-stimulating carotenoids. Consume cruciferous vegetables several times each week. The indoles in cabbage, broccoli, and other crucifers have potent antitumor activity and act as natural detoxifiers.

Consuming animal fats, primary sources of saturated fats, increases your risk for many kinds of cancer. Reduce saturated fat intake by limiting red meat, pork, and poultry. Eat more fish, especially those rich in omega-3 fatty acids such as salmon, tuna, and mackerel.

Avoid foods that contain antibiotics, hormones, artificial sweeteners, colorings, or harmful additives. Eat organically grown produce or use a commercial fruit and vegetable wash to remove pesticides and waxes. When grilled or cooked at high temperatures, meat forms potent carcinogens that may be harmful to lung tissue.

Step Nine: Consider Dietary Supplementation
Here's something to really think about: A study of late-stage patients with small cell lung cancer who were treated with

chemotherapy and antioxidants cocktail lived longer than patients who underwent chemotherapy without antioxidants. In the past twenty years, I have employed both traditional and non-traditional nutritional therapies and here's what I've found: patients that take dietary supplements in support of a healthy diet experience the most profound health benefits. I have come to realize that it is almost impossible for cancer patients to eat right, consistently, every day. If the body doesn't get what it needs to heal, it won't heal. Conversely, if the body gets what it needs to fight cancer, it will!

Dosage of dietary supplements need to be adjusted based on individual needs which can vary considerably based on medical condition, illness history, prescription medication, dietary habits, and lifestyle factors. Because dietary supplements can have pharmacological activity, you should inform all medical providers who are responsible for your care about your vitamin or herbal regimen. I will first discuss a few supplements that everyone with lung cancer needs to know about.

Two separate studies of high-risk groups (smokers and asbestos workers) concluded that high dose beta-carotene supplementation promoted cancer growth. Although researchers did not consider that beta-carotene readily oxidizes in these toxic environments, we are learning that supplementing with high doses of individual nutrients, even plant chemicals, may create imbalance and be detrimental to cancer outcome. That is specifically why a plant-based diet and whole foods nutrition supplement is ideal. Based on many other studies, it appears the safest way to take beta-carotene or other antioxidants is in combination with other antioxidants. For maximum cancer preventive effects, choose a supplement that contains a mixture of carotenoids, not just beta-carotene alone. The take home message is simple: Avoid synthetic beta-carotene if you are a smoker.

N-acetyl cysteine is also an important supplement to discuss.

Glutathione is a powerful antioxidant, immune stimulator, and regulator of cell division. Glutathione can protect the liver from harmful toxins. Researchers are divided on how well glutathione is absorbed and studies have shown that whey protein or 500 mg of ascorbic acid can be used to sufficiently raise glutathione levels. Additionally, animal experiments showed that the concentrates of whey proteins exhibited anticarcinogenic and anticancer activity. For these reasons, vitamin C-rich foods or whey protein may be the best ways to get additional glutathione into your diet. N-acetyl cysteine (NAC) is a component of glutathione. Both animal and human studies of NAC have shown it is a potential cancer-fighting agent. NAC, in combination with ascorbic acid, protected against lung cancer development in mice. NAC has also exhibited antiangiogenesis properties (decreased blood supply to tumors). 500 to 1,000 mg per day is a suggested dosage. NAC may interfere with cisplatin, so avoid if this platinum-based chemotherapy is part of your treatment plan.

Melatonin is a neurohormone that can modulate immunity. Melatonin reduced cytotoxic damage to bone marrow and lymphoid tissues, and stimulated suppressed bone marrow. Animal studies demonstrated melatonin's anticancer effect on lung cancer and hormonally related cancers such as breast, prostate, and ovarian cancers. Survival rates increased when melatonin was used with interleukin-2 and interferon cancer treatments. Dosage ranges from 3 to 20 mg per day and melatonin levels should be monitored by a health care professional during administration of this supplement.

Selenium was studied in a randomized, double-blind, placebo controlled trial and researchers concluded that the death rate from lung cancer was significantly less in the selenium group than the placebo group. Therapeutic levels of selenium range 100-200 mcg per day; however, I recommend a whole food version of selenium. Simply eat two to three Brazil nuts per day to receive a hefty dose of natural selenium surrounded by other cancer-fighting plant chemicals found in nuts.

Omega-3 fatty acids protect against cancer by creating a slippery environment so that cancer cells can't spread. The best source of omega-3 fatty acids is cold water fish. In order to get enough omega-3 fatty acids into the diet, in addition to consuming a couple of fish meals per week, you will need to take a fish oil supplement. As I previously mentioned, you will want to look for a therapeutic brand of fish oil to ensure your product is free from mercury, pesticides and other contaminants. Your fish oil supplements should provide you with a daily dose of at least 240-360 mg of EPA and 100-240 mg of DHA. Fish oil does cause the blood to thin, so be sure to inform your doctor prior to surgery or if you are on a blood-thinning medication.

Dietary supplements can help with detoxification as well. When people have cancer, their cellular protection systems are out of balance due to exposure to chemicals, poor dietary choices, and the debilitating effects of illness. In an effort to counterbalance cellular destruction and assist the body's natural detoxification processes, nutritional supplements can be used in combination with a whole foods diet and a juicing regimen.

Many nutrients are needed to support the function of organs directly involved in whole body cleansing. For example, psyllium husk and other soluble fibers, along with fructooligosaccharides, acidophilus culture, and L-glutamine promote a healthy gastrointestinal tract. You can support liver health with vitamins A, C, and E, and selenium, zinc, calcium, L-cysteine, and milk thistle. Kidney health is supported by vitamins A, C, B6, and the minerals magnesium and potassium. Dandelion and parsley have natural diuretic properties.

The toxic side effects of cisplatin, a type of chemotherapy often used in lung cancer treatment, can be reduced with the intake of gingko, milk thistle and quercetin.

Obviously, there are many choices to consider when taking dietary supplements to support your cancer treatment regimen.

Where should you start? There are two foundational supplements that I personally take and recommend to everyone: 1) a whole food phytochemical supplement called Juice Plus+ (www.juiceplusmed.com); and 2) a therapeutic grade fish oil (Carlson and Nordic Naturals are good brands). These food-based supplements are safe and clinically proven to be effective.

Beyond those two supplements, please visit with a health care professional who is familiar with oncology nutrition and complementary medicine. Seeking the advice of a training professional prior to taking dietary supplements, especially higher levels of individual nutrients, is important so that you take the adequate dose of nutrients and avoid imbalance or potentially dangerous interactions with medications.

Chapter 8

Protocel® for Lung Cancer – Tanya Harter Pierce, MA, MFCC

One thing I have learned with certainty over ten years of investigation is that there are *many* ways to cure cancer! All of the runs, walks and other fund-raising events to 'find the cure' are simply perpetuating a deadly misconception. Well, two misconceptions actually. The first misconception is that there is only one cure to find, and the second is that there exist no effective cures right now. The conundrum is that virtually all of the really good cures are *outside* mainstream medicine. This means they are labeled 'alternative' and the average cancer patient will never hear about them.

This chapter is about one of those effective alternative cures. It is called Protocel®, and is a single-product approach that comes in the form of a brown liquid formula. It can be purchased without a doctor's prescription, yet has been powerful enough to bring about countless complete cancer cures over the past two decades, often as a stand-alone approach by itself. In fact, many of the recovery stories have been so astounding that this treatment has sometimes been misconstrued as a 'magic bullet'.

Protocel® is one of the least expensive methods for treating cancer that exists anywhere, costing the average cancer patient between $70 and $140 per month, depending on dosage needs. Yet, in the bigger scheme of things, only a small percentage of the public has ever heard about Protocel®. Unfortunately, the American Cancer Society, National Cancer Institute and Food and Drug Administration have all played a role in keeping it that way.

Who am I? I am the author of a book called *Outsmart Your*

Cancer: Alternative Non-Toxic Treatments That Work. The first edition came out in 2004 and an updated expanded second edition was released in 2009. Unlike the other esteemed writers of chapters in this book, I do not have a medical degree, and if anyone had told me before August of 2001 that I would write a book about cancer treatments, I would have fallen off my chair. At that time, I was a newly retired Marriage, Family, Child Counselor. I had just closed down my counseling practice to work on a self-help book on another subject, and had already started that writing project. Suddenly, a family member of mine was diagnosed with cancer. He was not given a good prognosis for long-term recovery through mainstream medicine, and was interested in finding out what alternative options might be available to him. So I stopped everything I was doing and started looking into possible options outside of mainstream medicine to see if I could help.

I thought this detour would take a few months of my time at most and that I would get back to my original book project. But as I came across more and more information about non-toxic alternative cancer treatments, I was astounded at how many had *better* track records at curing cancer than mainstream medicine. I was also surprised that many of them had been developed by highly respected physicians or scientists such as microbiologists, chemists, physicists and the like.

I then started talking to cancer patients who had used alternative methods successfully and their stories confirmed that the approaches I'd been reading about really did work in real life. Many of the recovered patients I spoke with had been given up on by conventional medicine and told by their oncologist to go home and get their affairs in order. It was often *after* that dire pronouncement that they finally tried alternative medicine.

My first reaction was, "Why hadn't I heard about any of these curative approaches before?" And, "Why weren't oncologists and cancer clinics everywhere using them?" For goodness sakes, it felt like I was discovering the existence of numerous *underground* treatments that hundreds or even thousands of cancer patients had used to cure themselves! How could there be effective treatments that most cancer patients never hear about? There was something very wrong with this picture.

As the stack of books and other printed material on my desk got higher and higher and I became ever more intrigued by the recovery cases I was coming across, I decided to put my first book project on indefinite hold and write about alternative cancer treatments instead. I wrote *Outsmart Your Cancer* from the vantage point of an investigative reporter presenting the history and science behind numerous different non-toxic treatment methods. I interviewed scores of cancer survivors and wrote up their cases. And, when the second edition came out, I included an audio CD in every book that presented twelve ordinary people telling their alternative treatment recovery stories in their own words.

In the process, I also became an expert on the Protocel® formula and *Outsmart Your Cancer* quickly became the definitive source of printed information on this particular approach. Soon, I was receiving hundreds of phone calls and emails every year from cancer patients or doctors throughout the US and other countries who wanted to learn more about it.

As already mentioned, there are still no 'magic bullets' out there. But many of the recovery cases I have come across using either Protocel® or one of the other powerful alternative methods I describe in my book are clean, straightforward recoveries that can only be attributed to the alternative method used. And, with one out of every four deaths in America now a cancer death, we don't need to set our sights as high as a magic bullet. Simply having options that work *much better* than what oncologists are prescribing now would be a great improvement and could save many thousands of lives. It is no secret that conventional treatments for cancer today are *not* showing an acceptable track record.

For instance, if we look at current official statistics for lung cancer patients treated with conventional methods, we find that:

- A whopping sixty percent of all lung cancer patients die within the first year after they are diagnosed.
- About half of the remaining forty percent die within the second year after they are diagnosed, leaving only 20% living at the two-year mark.
- A few years later, just five years after diagnosis, only 12 to 15% of all lung cancer patients are still alive. But this does *not* mean those 12 to 15% are cured. Many of them still have cancer and succumb to their illness shortly after the 5-year mark. Thus, the real overall cure rate for lung cancer using mainstream medicine, including those where the cancer was caught very early, is most likely *less than ten out of every 100 patients.*
- And if we look at those lung cancer patients whose cancer has already metastasized beyond the lungs and localized lymph nodes when they are first diagnosed, official statistics state that those cases have only a 2.1% chance of living 5 years or more. Unfortunately, official statistics also show that at least 40% (nearly half) of all lung cancer patients already have distant metastasized cancer when they are first diagnosed. This means that, in the realm of conventional treatment, *nearly half of all lung cancer patients face only about a 2% chance of being alive 5 years after they are diagnosed!*

These statistics are dismal and especially disturbing since they apply to the most commonly diagnosed type of cancer in our country.

I'm not saying we should throw out conventional treatments altogether. They are sometimes critically needed, and surgery alone can be curative occasionally if the cancer is caught extremely early. But it is time for the public to know that there are other options, too. Options that can often produce a full recovery when conventional treatment can't.

Some of the approaches I have written about in my book are nutritional/dietary methods, some are herbal, and others are simply unique treatments that don't fall under any particular category. Protocel® is one of the unique treatments. Developed by a brilliant American chemist named Jim Sheridan, Protocel® can in some ways be described best by what it is not. It is not a vitamin or mineral formula, it is not herbal, and it is not homeopathic. Protocel®'s ingredients are listed as "a proprietary blend of Tetrahydroxyquinone, Rhodizonic Acid, sodium, potassium, Croconic Acid, Triquinoyl, Pyrocatechol, Leuconic Acid, mineral and trace elements, including copper." None of the ingredients by themselves have significant anti-cancer effects, but when it comes to Protocel®, the whole is greater than the parts. When put together in just the right way, this unique formula works like a catechol to block the energy production of cancer cells without harming any normal healthy cells of the body. Multiple toxicity tests have proven it to be less toxic than an aspirin a day.

Protocel® is so safe, in fact, it has been given to toddlers and other young children, as well as self-administered by seniors in their eighties or nineties. I have spoken to cancer patients on fixed budgets with only Medicare health insurance who are using it to treat their cancer because it is so affordable and no other expensive supplements are needed along with it. I have also communicated with people who are confined to wheelchairs or who are vision or hearing impaired using Protocel® for their cancer because it is so easy to use. For example, here are two case stories that show just how good an option Protocel® can be for some people who are limited in their treatment options.

Case Story #1 – Sara (Florida)

Sara was diagnosed in June of 2003 with lung cancer at the age of 82. She had been a smoker for 55 years, had emphysema as well as COPD, and had also experienced bouts of bronchitis off and on for many years. During a routine appointment with her lung specialist for breathing difficulties, a mass was seen on an x-ray in her right lung. A PET scan was ordered and the lung specialist thought she had lung cancer. Sara was sent to an oncologist, another PET scan was done, and the oncologist also diagnosed lung cancer. From looking at the scans, the tumor appeared to be a little larger than a grape.

Sara's doctors recommended chemotherapy and radiation, but she didn't want to have anything to do with those treatments at her age, considering the other health challenges she was already dealing with. She'd heard about Protocel® a few years earlier and the following is how she describes her decision to use it instead of conventional methods.

Just a few years ago, I heard about Protocel® through a friend who was discussing it with my daughter. I didn't pay too much attention to it at the time, although it was a remarkable story we never forgot. My friend had been diagnosed with breast cancer and was to go in for a mastectomy to have both breasts removed. She had only been on Protocel® for two weeks prior to her scheduled surgery, but when she went in and they did preliminary scans prior to the mastectomy, they couldn't find anything. The cancer was gone. So they cancelled her surgery. They had no explanation, other than that she'd been taking Protocel®. Puzzling to everyone, but how attention getting! What a miracle. We never forgot her story.

But in 2003, when I was diagnosed with lung cancer, I was still skeptical. My daughter is the one who got me to take Protocel®. She told me if I would take it that she would quit smoking. Well, since I'd been a smoker for 55 years and never wanted this to happen to my daughter, I immediately agreed. And as it turns out, we both turned out to be big winners.

When the PET scan showed the extent of the lung cancer, my doctors wanted me to do radiation and chemotherapy, and I told them I would do neither. Instead, I would be using Protocel®. And being 82 at the time, my doctors knew me well enough to know it was futile to try to get me to change my mind. So they said, "Well, we'll see what this does."

Sara ordered the Protocel® for herself and took a quarter teaspoonful of the liquid four times a day, every five and a half hours. She took no other supplements and used no other treatments whatsoever except for her nebulizer that she'd already been using for her emphysema and COPD. She first started taking the Protocel® in July of 2003 and continued taking it every day. In September of the same year, she had her first PET scan follow-up. The results showed that the mass in her lung was still there and the same size as when she was diagnosed. But the fact that it had not grown and no new metastases had developed, seemed encouraging.

Just two months later, in November, another scan showed that the tumor was getting smaller and still no new tumors had developed. With that encouragement, Sara just kept taking the Protocel® four times every day and otherwise living a normal life. In 2004, she reached the 'all-clear' point when x-rays showed her lungs to be free of all masses. Her doctor couldn't understand it and apologized for scaring her, thinking she must have been misdiagnosed. (Sara never told him she had been using an alternative treatment all those months.)

Sara kept taking the Protocel® until she'd been on it for about a year after her all-clear point. Then she stopped and has not taken it since. She says that while she was on the Protocel® she had absolutely no ill effects at all and also caught no colds and felt very good and energetic.

Sara's last scans were on March 18, 2009 and she is delighted to report that they still showed no sign of cancer. At the time of this writing in December of 2010, it is seven and a half years after she was diagnosed with lung cancer and refused all conventional treatment. Sara is 89 years old now and feels well and full of vigor!

Case Story #2 – Arch (South Carolina)

In June of 2006, 80-year-old Arch was getting a routine chest x-ray when a spot was discovered in his right lung. In Arch's own words:

We had all kinds of trouble getting appointments for follow-up, so it was late July before I got a biopsy on the lung spot. They told me it was 'non-small cell carcinoma'. CT and PET scans showed something suspicious in my neck and at the base of my tongue also. The mass on my neck was biopsied in August and was a carcinoma of the same type as in the lung. [It appeared to be metastasized lung cancer to a distant lymph node.]

I spent most of one day with a panel of specialists at a medical center who went over the whole thing. They didn't want to commit, but the general consensus was that I had only a 5 to 15% chance of a cure and a life expectancy of 3 to 4 years. Surgery on the lung was not advised. I questioned my doctor about whether we could cure cancer in the lung by any means other than surgery and he said reluctantly, "No, you really can't." All in all, it wasn't too encouraging.

Various doctors kept looking for whatever was at the base of my tongue, but it wasn't until late September that they found a tonsil that just didn't look right. In October, I had surgery on the neck and the tonsil. That wasn't a lot of fun. Starting in November, I got radiation to the lung and to the neck and shoulder 5 days a week. I made them stop the neck and shoulder part early because they were burning me to a 'crispy critter' and I couldn't take it anymore.

Now to the Protocel® part. My doctor gave me a copy of Tanya Pierce's book Outsmart Your Cancer, *and suggested I study the information about Protocel®. Based on that, I began taking Formula 50 in late August. The cancer on my neck, which was easy to see, got noticeably smaller during the 6 weeks on Protocel® before surgery. The surgeon had told me that it was about 6 cm long before I started on the Protocel®, but the pathologist found only a 1 cm carcinoma in the yellowish jelly-like material removed during surgery.*

I had CT scans first every three months, then every 6 months. All have shown no cancer, only some scarring in the lung. So I said, "Is it gone?" My doctor said, "As far as I can tell, it's gone. There's nothing there but a little scar tissue."

So I felt that the Protocel® took my cancer away! It's true that I did have some radiation to my right lung and head and neck area at first. But I stopped them short of the amount they wanted to give me. And my doctor said that lung cancer cannot be cured with anything other than surgery, meaning that he assumed it would be coming back. But the spot in my lung and the tumors in my neck and throat have not come back and it is now December of 2010, four and a half years after I was diagnosed. Last month, I got another CT scan of my head and whole trunk, and I'm still all-clear! I haven't done any treatment of any kind other than Protocel® since my surgery.

At my lowest point in all this, among many low points, I had lost about 30 pounds, had lost my sense of taste, and was very, very tired. I'm a lot better now and struggling not to get too fat. I'm also still taking Protocel®. It's so easy to do and so inexpensive, I think anybody with cancer ought to take it!

In Arch's case, his lung cancer was metastasized and, though he underwent some surgery and radiation, most cancer experts would agree that he would have shown signs of recurrence by now if conventional treatment was all that he had done. Plus, a panel of oncologists proclaimed that he only had a life expectancy of 3 to 4 years. It has now been four and a half years since that prognosis, and Arch is not only still alive, but shows no evidence of cancer anywhere!

Arch's story is also particularly interesting because the pathologist's report after his surgery described a tumor reduced in size from its original measurement and surrounded by a "yellowish jelly-like material". This jelly-like material is consistent with how Protocel® causes malignant tumors to break down through the process of lysing. In fact, one of the most common lysing symptoms that cancer patients using Protocel® report is that they see either clear, yellowish, or white mucousy material coming out of their body that is the consistency of egg whites. What they are seeing is the broken-down cancer cell debris being processed out of their body!

What Is Protocel® and How Was It Developed?

Protocel® has quite a colorful history. It was developed by an American man named James Vincent Sheridan, who was born into a Pennsylvania mining family in 1912, studied chemistry while on scholarship at Carnegie Tech in Pittsburgh, and went on to become a brilliant chemist.

As a young man, Jim Sheridan was both a top student and devoutly spiritual. Jim knew he had a good mind and, in his early teens, he prayed to God that he would be able to use his intellect to help mankind. He even prayed to be able to help find a cure for cancer some day, which was certainly *not* an ordinary thing for a teenage boy to do! For Sheridan, it wasn't his ego at play. He truly wanted to be of service to his fellow man. As if in answer to his prayers, during his late teens and early twenties, Jim experienced a series of auspicious events that seemed to lead him in the direction of service to his fellow man that he was seeking.

One of these events occurred on September 6, 1936, after he'd been studying biochemistry in college for a number of years. On this day, while he was taking an afternoon nap, Jim experienced a very unusual dream. Much of what he had already learned about cell functioning was confirmed by a sort of vision that he had in the dream. This vision also helped him to understand even more than he'd been taught in college about the oxygen reduction or 'redox' system of cell respiration. (NOTE: The term 'cell respiration' should not be confused with breathing. It refers to the process by which cells produce and distribute energy for themselves.) The dream revealed to Jim how to alter the pathway of energy production in cancer cells in a controlled way that could result in a cure for people suffering from this dreaded disease.

Jim Sheridan was profoundly affected by this dream and felt he'd been given an understanding of how to cure cancer. He started working immediately on how to incorporate what he learned from the dream to produce a practical treatment for cancer. Three years later, in 1939, he bought his first mice so that he could start testing the early versions of his formula.

It took Sheridan many years of hard work and trial and error to develop his formula fully. Overall, he worked on it from the late 1930s until the early 1990s. Much of that time, especially in the beginning, he was working in his spare time. At first, he was employed full-time as a chemist at Dow Chemical Company. He worked at Dow Chemical from 1935 to 1946. Then, in the early 1950s, Sheridan obtained a private grant to work at the Detroit Institute of Cancer Research (which later became the Michigan Cancer Foundation). Here, he was able to improve his liquid cancer treatment in a formal laboratory environment. Later, in the 1960s, Sheridan worked on his project for a few years at the Battelle Institute in Columbus, Ohio. Battelle was an organization that commonly tested new chemo agents for the National Cancer Institute and was officially recognized for animal testing. By 1983 Sheridan finally had a formula that could consistently cure about 80% of the laboratory mice with cancer that he treated.

During the early years, Sheridan called his formula "Entelev®". It was later called "Cancell®" before finally being renamed "Protocel®". Sheridan kept taking steps to have his formula studied by the various top cancer research organizations in the US, but his efforts to get official studies performed on it were blocked at every turn. This is the short version of the history and readers can go to *Outsmart Your Cancer* for many more in-depth details about how this effective cancer treatment was developed and later how it was actively obstructed by the ACS, NCI, and FDA between 1953 and 1992.

How Does Protocel® Work?

To understand the theory behind Jim Sheridan's formula, we start with the concept that all cancer cells primarily use an *anaerobic* cell respiration process called 'glycolysis' to produce energy for themselves. This is different from all healthy cells of the body, which primarily use an *aerobic* process that utilizes oxygen for energy production.

Anaerobic cell respiration is limited and much less efficient than aerobic cell respiration. Some normal cells of the body, such as muscle cells, may use anaerobic cell respiration at times for short periods under certain conditions. However, it is important to understand that any human cell which *only* uses anaerobic energy production all the time is an unhealthy or abnormal cell. In other words, it is a cell that has become so damaged it can no longer function normally and must rely on anaerobic energy production alone. Cancer cells fall into this category.

Exactly how Protocel® works on the cellular level is quite complicated, but two simple concepts are sufficient to understand. Firstly, Protocel® directly kills cancer cells by causing them to fall apart, or 'lyse'. Secondly, the way that Protocel® causes cancer cells to lyse is by biochemically interfering with their production of ATP (adenosine triphosphate).

Normal healthy cells that use aerobic functioning are not negatively impacted by Protocel® because they are very efficient at producing energy and have more than one biochemical pathway they can use to do so. But cancer cells are limited to the less efficient pathway of glycolysis, and it is this limitation that allows Protocel® to block their energy production enough to give them trouble. When about 10 to 15% of the ATP production in a cancer cell is blocked, this lowers the capacitance, or potential, of the cell. (Most lay people understand the term 'voltage' better, which is close enough.)

Because the glycolysis pathway for producing energy is not very efficient, cancer cells operate on a minimum energy level and sustain a lower voltage than normal healthy cells. The slight reduction in voltage that Protocel® causes shifts the cancer cells' energy downward to a point *below the minimum amount of energy that cancer cells need to keep their cell membranes intact*. In other words, cancer cells throughout the body are deprived of their energy in a slow but consistent way when people use Protocel® until the cancer cells no longer have enough energy to hold their cell membranes together. At this point, the cancer cells literally start to fall apart, or burst. In the science of biology, this process of bursting is called 'lysing'. It doesn't happen overnight, but is a gradual process that slowly and systematically brings about cancer regression, in many cases until the cancer is completely eliminated and never comes back.

Compared to chemotherapy or radiation, Protocel® works slowly on tumors. That is because it is *not* a toxic poison and was designed to cause cancer breakdown at a rate that a person's body can easily handle. Keep in mind, also, that this treatment is sold as a dietary supplement and its distributors make no claims as to its effectiveness against cancer. It is a self-administered approach, and there are no doctors who have chosen to become experts in its use. But this is primarily because, in most US states, doctors cannot legally prescribe any cancer treatment that is not approved by the FDA and sanctioned by their state medical board. Having said that, I have heard numerous cancer patients tell me that their doctor was the one who suggested they buy my book and consider Protocel® for their cancer.

Here are more cases that show various people's experiences using Protocel® for lung cancer, including when the cancer was metastasized at the time of diagnosis.

Case Story # 3 – Cindy (Kansas)

In May of 2007, 59-year-old Cindy started having pain in her back and experiencing shortness of breath. She thought she had pulled a muscle and went to her doctor to get checked. She was also coughing a lot, so the doctor ordered an x-ray of her lungs. The x-ray showed "a big spot" on her right lung and Cindy was referred to a nearby hospital for a more definitive CT scan. This scan revealed more than just a spot – there was a sizable mass in Cindy's lung measuring 8 cm across. (Approximately 3 inches in diameter.) It turned out that this large mass was pressing on Cindy's windpipe and was the main cause of her labored breathing. Further examination revealed that the lung cancer had also metastasized to Cindy's adrenal glands. A needle biopsy through the lower back confirmed the diagnosis of 'small-cell lung cancer, stage IV'.

According to Cindy: *The doctor told us I could do some radiation to shrink the tumor that was pushing on my windpipe, causing the shortness of breath. What he didn't tell me, but told my husband in private, was that I only had 7 to 8 weeks to live and doing the radiation was only to help me breathe easier.*

In other words, Cindy's oncologist was simply recommending palliative treatment, knowing full well that it would not cure her. Cindy had smoked cigarettes for 45 years, since she was 14 years old. But it was still a shock to receive this diagnosis, especially given the short amount of time she was told she had to live. (7 to 8 weeks is hardly enough time to get one's affairs in order.) Here is how Cindy tells the rest of her story.

Dan, my husband of 27 years, was not going to let me die without a fight. He spent the next few days researching and reading everything he could about different cancer treatments. He found out about Protocel® and immediately started me on the regimen. I took 31 radiation treatments to the lung and started Protocel® after the first week of radiation. The doctor was very surprised when I didn't keep deteriorating and seemed to be healthy, considering my diagnosis. He decided I should go for the chemo. At this time we hadn't told him about my taking Protocel®.

I did do two intravenous chemo treatments (was told I needed four but I didn't like the harm it was doing me and the sickness), and two rounds of the oral chemo pills, which lasted about two months. Since the radiation was **not** directed at my adrenals, the very short-term chemo was the only mainstream treatment I got for the metastases to those glands. I had the usual side effects, but for some reason I wasn't affected as badly as others I had talked to.

After that first month, I did not do any other conventional treatment at all, and no surgery of any kind was ever done. I just kept taking the Protocel® every 6 hours. (Four times a day spaced out around the 24-hour clock with one of the doses in the middle of the night.)

About two months after starting Protocel®, I also heard about the benefits of apricot seeds and started eating those, too. I would put some seeds in a coffee grinder and add about a teaspoonful of the ground seed powder to my juice or smoothie every day. I didn't really change my diet much, just stopped eating sugar and sodas and drank more water. The only other supplements I took were a multi-vitamin and coral calcium.

Six months later, my cancer was not visible on scans anymore and I felt better than I ever had! When we told my cancer doctor about Protocel®, he said, "I don't know what you're doing, but whatever it is, keep doing it!" Later, I was told doctors couldn't endorse alternative ideas. But in a roundabout way, he did. He could tell something was making me well, because in the beginning he wasn't even going to recommend chemo. I was too far gone!

All the cancer disappeared from the scans, including the metastases to my adrenals. It has now been three and a half years since I was diagnosed and still no sign of cancer.

I had two friends diagnosed shortly after I was, one with the same type of cancer as mine. I got one friend started on Protocel®. She didn't do any conventional medical treatments. After six months her cancer *had shrunk and she was so excited. Then six months later I was called and told she had died. They also told me that shortly after finding out her cancer had shrunk she quit taking the Protocel®. I was heartbroken. The other friend, the one that also had lung cancer, had seen how it had helped me get through the chemo and radiation side effects. She asked her doctor about taking Protocel® and was told to wait and see if the chemo helped. So she followed his orders, with me begging her to take Protocel® the whole time. After four chemo treatments, the cancer went to her brain and she died soon after.*

As already mentioned, Cindy had been a cigarette smoker since she was 14 years old. When she was diagnosed with lung cancer at age 59, she tried very hard to quit smoking, but found she just could not do it. Amazingly, she has continued to smoke since her diagnosis and through her entire use of Protocel®. Though this is *not* recommended for anyone trying to recover from cancer, Cindy continues to smoke and she takes Protocel® and apricot seeds every day to keep herself well.

After being diagnosed with a huge tumor in her lung, metastases to her adrenals, and having been given only 7 to 8 weeks to live, Cindy continues to feel fine with no sign of cancer three and a half years later!

Case Story # 4 – Carol (Pennsylvania)

Carol is a remarkable woman with another impressive story. She is 65 years old, and has had what most people would agree was not an easy life. She is diabetic and takes Metformin for that condition. She also has battled degenerative osteoarthritis for 24 years. Though she can walk and get around, there are periods when she suffers a lot of pain in her joints. On top of that, Carol was diagnosed with schizophrenia when she was in her twenties and takes psychiatric drugs for that condition. She says the schizophrenia has really caused a lot of ups and downs in her life and, though she learned to function well enough most of the time and has been active in her church, she finally had to go on disability and give up working a regular job.

Carol was married for almost 30 years, but then her husband died and she has been a widow living alone with no children for the past 10 years. Even so, Carol is a positive-minded person and not inclined to complain.

Over eight years ago, when Carol was 57, she noticed an enlargement in her abdomen and went to the doctor. An examination was performed and she was given a chest x-ray. The x-ray showed some masses in her lung. After that, a needle was inserted through her breast for a biopsy and the diagnosis came back 'non-small cell lung cancer, stage III'. To see if the tumors could be surgically removed, a camera device was inserted to view the cancer. Afterward, Carol's doctor said that her cancer was in the cradle of the heart area, which meant that surgery would be too risky and was not recommended. Chemotherapy and radiation *were* recommended, however.

But when Carol asked about the effectiveness of the chemo and radiation treatments, the doctor himself admitted that most patients taking chemotherapy and radiation live only about ten months. So Carol decided to decline all conventional treatment. She had heard about Protocel® from a friend, and decided to try that instead. According to Carol: *It took courage because I really didn't know if it would work or not. But my only option was that I would be dead in about ten months anyway.* The only other things Carol took along with the Protocel® were an enzyme supplement and an herb called paw paw, both supplements known to be compatible with Protocel®.

It is now almost nine years since Carol's oncologist told her that the best conventional medicine could do for her would most likely be to give her ten months! She kept going back to her doctor over the years for tests and scans and says that the Protocel®, paw paw and enzymes made all her tumors shrink in size and have prevented the cancer from traveling to other places in her body. Carol still has tumors, which may be benign masses at this point. Whatever they are, their growth appears to be controlled. Her doctor says she is amazing and finds her case very interesting.

Because of Carol's various conditions and all the drugs she has to take for those conditions, she has often missed her doses of Protocel® or been late in taking them. This may well be the main reason some masses have not completely resolved. She also didn't know that eating sugar would feed her cancer and work against the Protocel®. Since Carol has a strong sweet tooth, she has continued to eat sweets all these years. She also didn't know that she could increase her dose of Protocel® if the cancer wasn't completely going away, since some people do need a higher dose.

Thus, Carol's use of Protocel® has not been optimal. But given all the challenges Carol has had to deal with, it is truly commendable that she has been able to effectively control her cancer with no help from anyone else and while on a disability budget. She has shown remarkable courage and resourcefulness given the fact that her oncologist told her she would likely not live longer than 10 months, even with all the conventional treatment he had to offer her.

Happily, thanks to Protocel®, that was almost 9 years ago and Carol is still living a normal life!

Case Story #5 – Walt (California)

In May of 2008, 89-year-old Walt was rushed to the hospital. He'd been strong and healthy all his life. In fact, previous to this, the last time he was in a hospital as a patient was in 1958! Though not deaf, Walt suffers from hearing loss and can only hear people talking to him up close if they speak clearly. He often has trouble understanding doctors who speak fast or have any type of foreign accent. This condition has played a role in his general avoidance of doctors for much of his life.

Leading up to May of 2008, Walt had been feeling that his energy was low and he had been coughing off and on for about 6 months. But he didn't think much of it and figured he was probably just catching a cold. Suddenly, he felt a strong pain and grabbed his chest. His daughter was with him at the time and she thought he was having a heart attack. Walt was rushed to emergency where tests were done, including an x-ray. Afterward, the emergency room doctor came out to Walt's daughter and said, "The upper portion of your dad's left lung has collapsed... AND he has cancer."

This was a shock to Walt and his family, but there was no questioning the reality of it a week later after he was referred to a lung specialist. A CT scan was performed and a biopsy procedure done. Next, Walt saw an oncologist to discuss the scan and biopsy reports and was given the official diagnosis of 'Squamous Cell Cancer, Stage III'. The tests showed a single mass measuring 3 by 5 cm, or about 1.25 inches wide by 2 inches long. No other tumors or metastases were found.

Walt's daughter asked the oncologist what had caused the cancer and the doctor replied it had probably resulted from Walt's cigarette smoking, since he had smoked from the young age of 13 until he was 45. But he'd stopped at that point, which was 44 years prior to his cancer diagnosis! However, the oncologist still thought his smoking was the most likely cause and also said that Walt's particular lung cancer was slow-growing. When asked about a prognosis, Walt was given a better answer than many lung cancer patients receive. The oncologist thought that Walt could possibly live about two and a half years if he did no treatment at all because his cancer was slow-growing.

Walt's oncologist then explained to him that, at age 89, he was too old for surgery. But the doctor did suggest treatment and said, "We're going to put you on chemotherapy and give you radiation at the same time." Walt was nervous about the recommended treatment and questioned the radiation in particular because the mass was so close to his heart. To that, the doctor replied, "Don't worry about it, we're really good at this."

Walt was stubborn and declined the chemo and radiation anyway. The oncologist then made a secondary recommendation, which was that Walt could take an oral chemo pill and see if that worked for him. But when Walt and his daughter found out that this medication would cost $4,000 a month for just 30 pills, he declined that, too.

Walt's daughter had already heard about Protocel® from a friend, and Walt decided to try that instead. He rejected all conventional treatment and started taking the Protocel® formula in June of 2008, one month after he'd been diagnosed with lung cancer. Because Walt did not sleep a lot at night and knew that Protocel® was most effective when spaced out evenly around the 24-hour clock, he simply took one-quarter teaspoonful in water every six hours (at 6 am, 12 noon, 6 pm, and midnight) every single day. He also started a B-vitamin supplement and took vitamin D. That was all Walt did to control his cancer. He didn't change his diet much, just reduced his sugar intake.

Six weeks after starting Protocel®, Walt went back for another CT scan and was told that the tumor in his lung was just a little bigger than it had been before. Walt was not swayed by this because 6 weeks is often not long enough to see tumor reduction with this approach, and he kept taking the Protocel®. He got another x-ray in November of 2008 (five months after starting Protocel®). This time, the mass in his lung was definitely smaller and no new masses were showing.

Through 2009, Walt avoided going to the doctor and just lived his life normally until December, when he went back in for another x-ray. Once again, the tumor was smaller than the last time and no new masses were apparent. Walt's oncologist said to him, "Well, you're doing great Walt! What are you doing now?" So he finally told his doctor about the Protocel®. His doctor replied, "Keep doing what you're doing!"

The problem of Walt's lung having partially collapsed had not been of much concern to the doctors all along, and the December

'09 x-ray showed that the affected lung had almost completely re-inflated by itself, with only a small part of the top of his lung not quite having returned to normal yet. Interestingly, Walt had also had a nasty looking mole on his arm about the size of a penny that was very black. After starting Protocel®, that mole gradually went from black to a light tan and continues to remain light in color.

As of this writing in December of 2010, Walt is 91 years old and is still taking Protocel®. It is now two and a half years after he was diagnosed. His last x-ray just two months ago showed that his tumor appears to have stabilized in size – not smaller but not bigger either – and there are still no signs of metastases! Though Walt has not completely gotten his tumor to go away, he has successfully been able to stabilize his cancer and suffers no ill effects from either the cancer or from the Protocel® he is taking. Most importantly, he is able to live a normal life and does not have to spend much time in doctors' offices, undergoing difficult tests or treatments. According to Walt's daughter, he feels good, though now that he is 91 he isn't as active as he used to be and doesn't go outside and do his gardening quite as much as before!

Case Story #6 – Jon (Pennsylvania)

Jon is 67 years old and manages his own health food store. He also feels great and lives an extremely healthy lifestyle. But almost four years ago, things were quite a different story.

In March of 2007, Jon began experiencing chest pain and shortness of breath. He went to the hospital thinking he was having a heart attack. As it turned out, his heart was not the problem. He was diagnosed as having a gallbladder attack and immediate surgical removal of the gallbladder was recommended. Also, a chest x-ray showed a spot on one of his lungs. Jon was referred to an oncologist and after a needle biopsy was performed, he was diagnosed with lung cancer. Jon's oncologist was adamant that he immediately needed both gallbladder surgery *and* lung surgery, followed by chemotherapy and radiation for his cancer. The oncologist told Jon that if he did not go through the recommended surgery and follow-up treatments, *he would be dead in six months.*

But Jon did not feel the recommended treatments were right for him. He already had an action plan in case he ever got cancer, which was to use alternative therapies to heal himself, and he knew a man who was doing well on Protocel® for a rare type of carcinoid lung cancer that had been caused by exposure to Agent Orange in Vietnam.

So, Jon declined all conventional treatment. He had learned about gallbladder cleanses and did repeated cleanses for about two months to heal his gallbladder. He also read a lot of books on alternative cancer treatments and eventually settled on Protocel® with some other supportive supplements and cleanses (all the while making sure that he only chose supplements that were considered compatible with Protocel®). Jon also switched to a raw vegan diet. He said the first three months were the hardest because he gave up all the foods he was addicted to, like breads and sugars. He also did coffee enemas.

At first, right after his diagnosis, Jon could only walk a short distance before the pain in his lung and shortness of breath stopped him. But he kept doing the program he had developed for himself, including taking Protocel® four times every day because he wholeheartedly believed that his body could heal itself. After a few months, Jon could walk much farther without pain. But he still felt a tugging discomfort in his lung whenever he tried to breathe deeply. Eventually, that discomfort went away. His gallbladder normalized as well and it no longer caused him any problem.

It has been almost four years since Jon's oncologist told him he'd be dead in six months if he did not do surgery, chemotherapy and radiation for his cancer, and also since he was told he needed to have his gallbladder removed. Since declining all those treatments and taking charge of his own healing, he now runs 5 miles every day, looks 20 years younger than his true age according to everyone he meets, and feels better overall than he has ever felt in his life!

Jon never went back to the hospital to have any follow-up scans, so he cannot prove that his cancer is completely gone. On the other hand, one must wonder if follow-up scans are necessary in Jon's case, given how active, energetic and healthy he is, and given that a full four years have gone by with no conventional treatment used, not even surgery. And, since the original diagnosis was arrived at after a needle biopsy, he can definitely claim he had lung cancer.

Jon has obviously done something right, and he gives most of the credit to the Protocel® he took. He continues to take Protocel® along with some other health-supporting supplements and a good diet.

Case Story # 7 – Ruth (Michigan)

In April of 2006, Ruth was 66 years old when she developed pneumonia. X-rays revealed that she also had a large mass in her right lung. A month later, after more tests and a biopsy, Ruth was diagnosed with non-small cell lung cancer and her doctor's report listed the official diagnosis as 'adenocarcinoma of the right middle lobe, stage 1B, not smoking-induced'. (Ruth had never been a smoker, but did live around second-hand smoke for many years.) Immediate surgery was recommended and Ruth's oncologist said she'd probably also need follow-up chemotherapy and radiation treatments as well.

Ruth tells her story in the following description.

I heard about Protocel® from my sister-in-law who has a business in Cadillac, Michigan. There was a lady that had come into her business and shared her story about how she had cancer throughout her body (colon cancer metastasized to about six other areas) and took Protocel®

and was doing great.

I told my sister-in-law to order the Protocel® and the book Outsmart Your Cancer *on the Internet and started taking the Protocel® two weeks before my surgery. In the surgery, they removed 40% of the upper lobe and 10% of the middle lobe of my right lung. After the surgery, the doctor still thought I might have to do chemotherapy, but the lymph nodes they took out were all clear and I was worried about the damage chemo would do to me. So, the doctor didn't push the chemo because he said it didn't work well for my type of cancer anyway. But the oncologist made it clear that my cancer could come back anytime, so we'd have to watch it.*

I continued to take the Protocel® at home after the surgery. It made the pain much more bearable and I seemed to get much stronger. When I went back to my oncologist's office in September of that year, everyone was amazed at how good I looked and how well I was doing physically.

The first scans showed Ruth's tumor to be 2.3 cm in diameter, but by the time she went in for surgery in June, the mass had grown to 3.5 cm across. After the surgery, no evidence of cancer was left. At first, Ruth went back to her doctor every 6 months, then once a year. On her visit in June of '09, Ruth's oncologist wrote in her chart that she was "3 years disease-free". Her latest visit in July of 2010 showed her to be "4 years disease-free".

Ruth is now 70 years old and continues to remain very active. She paints, wallpapers, works in her flower garden and has lots of energy. She lives alone on a restricted budget with her only source of income being Social Security. She continues to take Protocel® to keep herself disease-free and once in a while she takes the herbal supplement, paw paw. She also takes vitamin D and some other supportive supplements for her bones.

In Ruth's case, there is a remote possibility that the surgery alone cured her, since her cancer was still localized when the surgery was done as far as the doctors could tell. However, her oncologist originally recommended that she follow the surgery with chemotherapy and radiation to make sure they got every last cancer cell. Without knowing about Protocel®, Ruth probably would have felt she had to do the conventional toxic follow-up treatments to keep her cancer from coming back. Since those treatments can have very negative side effects, who knows if she would be feeling so well today had she not been aware of a non-toxic therapy she could use instead!

Some important lessons can be learned from the above courageous people and their remarkable stories. One is that it is a good idea for any cancer patient to ask their oncologist directly what their chances for full recovery are if they go with conventional treatment alone (such as surgery, radiation and/or chemotherapy). As in Carol's case, her oncologist honestly admitted that most patients given chemotherapy and radiation for inoperable stage III lung cancer live only about ten months. Knowing this was valuable to Carol because it gave her the courage to try an alternative approach instead.

Patience and diligence when using an alternative method for cancer are also important because, as these cases illustrate, non-toxic approaches generally work more slowly on cancer than toxic therapies such as chemo or radiation. It is also critically important for anyone using an alternative method such as Protocel® to do their homework and look into what can and cannot be used along with the Protocel® approach. Various vitamins, minerals and herbs, and even some drugs or other alternative approaches may interfere with Protocel®'s action on the cellular level. Thus, it is important to look into how to use this liquid formula effectively if one wants to achieve the best possible results. (Some details about usage are listed in the upcoming pages of this chapter and many more details are presented in my book *Outsmart Your Cancer*.)

Last but not least, the benefit of knowing about a powerful non-toxic treatment that can be used as a follow-up to surgery instead of chemotherapy or radiation cannot be overstated. As the last testimonial illustrates, Ruth's cancer was caught early and may have been cured by her surgery alone. But it was only because she had heard about the effectiveness of Protocel® that she was able to decline the chemo and radiation follow-up treatments and therefore not take the risk of experiencing any of the life-threatening side effects those treatments might have caused.

Protocel® can be used for any type of cancer as long as it really is malignant cancer. (There is some question as to whether Protocel® will work for benign tumors and my own observation from talking to many people is that it does *not* work for truly benign tumors or pre-cancerous conditions such as DCIS that are not yet malignant.) In my book, I present real-life case stories of people who have used Protocel® for breast cancer, prostate cancer, stomach cancer, pancreatic cancer, kidney cancer, primary brain cancer, childhood leukemia, and melanoma, among others.

As with any treatment approach, the more advanced a person's illness is, the lower one's chances for full recovery tend to be. Even so, there have been a number of notable late-stage recoveries with this easy-to-use liquid formula. One that was particularly impressive was reported to me by a woman in Australia who had not found out she had breast cancer until it had already heavily metastasized to her bones. This woman's scans showed numerous lesions in her hips, legs, ribs, shoulder, spine and skull and she was in terrible pain. Her doctors performed surgery on her – not to take out the cancer, but simply to insert metal pins in her bones to keep them from crumbling. In fact, she lost a full three inches in height due to the bone damage she suffered from her extensive cancer metastases. This woman (who tells her story on the Audio CD at the back of my book) relied solely on Protocel®, since she knew that conventional treatments would be virtually useless for her situation. She chose to take it every four hours throughout the day and night. (Six times around the 24-hour clock.) The first year was very painful as her bones had to heal and she had to learn to walk again first with a walker, then with a cane. But this woman got back to full functioning and living a completely normal life again through her use of the Protocel® formula alone!

Obstructive Tactics and Misinformation

For many decades, the cancer industry has been in the business of obstructive tactics and misinformation. And it is a very effective business. In fact, it is quite easy to turn people away from a powerful cancer treatment or block it from being studied with just a few simple techniques.

With Protocel®, the first obstructive tactic occurred in late 1953. Jim Sheridan was working at the Detroit Institute of Cancer Research at the time and achieving such great results with his formula on laboratory mice that the Institute's director decided it was time to test the formula in human clinical trials. Other experts, including three oncologists from nearby hospitals, also looked at the data and agreed that it was time for human trials. But when the Detroit Institute's director informed the American Cancer Society of the intended trials, the ACS responded in a very bizarre way. They said they did not approve of the program because Jim Sheridan "had not proved that he owned the idea." This was a very strange response that had no apparent legal precedent. Nevertheless, the American Cancer Society somehow had the power to immediately halt the intended clinical trials. Jim Sheridan was then suspiciously fired from the Detroit Institute of Cancer Research. Even *more* suspicious was that Sheridan later learned that all the results of his research at the Institute had been burned!

But Sheridan did not give up. Between 1978 and 1980, he was able to get the NCI to finally agree to test his formula on laboratory mice. As is commonly the case, the NCI requested any information on special requirements it should know about to perform the animal tests. Sheridan complied by giving the NCI just three requirements. He said that: 1) the NCI should *not* inject the formula into the mice, but must administer it orally in water;

2) the NCI should make the test period at least 28 days because the formula did not make tumors disappear quite as fast as toxic chemo drugs; and 3) the NCI should not test the formula on mice with leukemia because mice with leukemia *always* die within 18 or 19 days and it would take just a little longer than that for his formula to work effectively.

What was supposed to happen next was that the results of the animal tests would then be forwarded to the FDA as a basis for considering human clinical trials. But what occurred instead was that Sheridan received a letter from the National Cancer Institute stating that his formula had been proved to be completely ineffective in the animal studies. When he looked into how the studies had been carried out, he discovered that the NCI had *ignored* all three of his specifications! They had injected his formula instead of administering it orally in water; they had used mice with leukemia rather than mice with any other type of cancer; and they had carried out the entire test in a mere 8 days rather than giving it the full 28 days. Of course, Sheridan called the NCI and requested that they repeat the animal tests according to his required protocol. They agreed to do the testing a second time, but unbelievably, they completely ignored his instructions again!

Jim Sheridan was never able to get the National Cancer Institute to test his formula correctly. Many people believe that the NCI deliberately chose to ignore Sheridan's instructions. Others believe the fiasco was just the result of an institution being entrenched in certain testing modes and unable to change their procedures. Whatever the reason, it worked out quite well for the obstruction of this cancer treatment because now the cancer industry can claim that animal studies performed by the NCI showed that Jim Sheridan's formula was ineffective. And if anyone searches for Protocel® on the NCI's official website, they will find the following statement:

studies showing its therapeutic effectiveness in animals have not been provided to the FDA.

What the NCI *does not say* on their website is that: 1) the results of all the incredibly positive animal studies done at the Detroit Cancer Institute were ignored by the ACS when clinical trials were sought and all the data was then suspiciously burned; and 2) the NCI failed to perform the animal tests correctly each time Sheridan's formula was submitted to them for evaluation.

Undaunted, Sheridan filed paperwork with the FDA in 1982 to try another way of getting his formula considered for clinical trials. The FDA did issue him an IND number. However, they also said that the study of his product had been put on "clinical hold" because he had not provided data assessing its toxicity. Though Sheridan had put his formula through a number of MLD (minimum lethal dose) tests on animals that proved it was non-toxic, he had not yet put it through an official LD-50 test through an FDA-approved laboratory. Unfortunately, every time Sheridan tried to do so, the laboratory refused to test his formula. It is believed that these FDA-approved labs were being pressured or threatened by the FDA into *not* testing his formula, and this turned out to be yet another very effective obstructive tactic.

Then, on November 13, 1990, the NCI agreed to test Sheridan's formula once more –this time on various cancer cell lines in vitro (not animal studies, but studies on cancer cells in containers). The results were excellent and, though the tests were only done over 48 hours, they showed that Sheridan's formula was highly effective against the eight different strains of cancer the NCI tested it on. (Graphs of these test results are presented in *Outsmart Your Cancer* using original data obtained from the NCI.) Jim Sheridan thought his formula might get formally studied now. Once again, however, he was shocked when he received a letter from the NCI stating that they were *not* planning to pursue his formula as a medical treatment. Sheridan was in his late seventies at this point and he was emotionally crushed.

Finally, Jim Sheridan's son, James E. Sheridan, decided to get involved. His son, a district court judge for the state of Michigan, phoned the NCI for an explanation of why they weren't going to pursue his father's formula. He spoke to Dr. Ven Narayanan, who was the head of drug testing for the NCI at the time. According to Judge Sheridan, Dr. Narayanan *agreed* that the in vitro tests showed his father's formula to be effective at killing cancer. But he then went on to say, "I could also obtain these results with chemotherapy, if I wanted to, but anything that would get results *this good* would be too toxic to humans!"

Judge Sheridan replied to Dr. Narayanan that the formula was *not* toxic and had been proven to be non-toxic by many MLD tests. But the NCI would only believe an LD-50 test done in an FDA-approved lab. Of course, the FDA had already effectively blocked all tests of that sort, so Sheridan did not have the paperwork to prove to the NCI that his treatment was non-toxic. In retrospect, both the FDA and the NCI appeared to be in collusion to make sure this cancer treatment did *not* get considered or tested in any meaningful way.

The last act of official suppression occurred on November 13, 1992, when a federal judge enforced an FDA injunction to stop all distribution of Sheridan's formula. (This injunction had first been issued in 1989, but not enforced for several years.) At that time, the formula was called Cancell® and had never been sold to anyone, but had only been *given away* to cancer patients for free. A retired businessman named Ed Sopcak had been producing and mailing the product out at his own expense for many years.

Sopcak later claimed that the FDA injunction was totally illegal because the FDA did not have a plaintiff (not one single person complained about the product), and also because there was never a hearing. Nevertheless, the FDA injunction effectively stopped all cancer patients from obtaining this effective non-toxic treatment.

After Congress passed the DSHEA Act in 1994, which took control over supplements away from the FDA, Sheridan's liquid formula was finally able to be reproduced as a dietary supplement in late 1999. This is when it was renamed Protocel®. An official LD-50 test was requested again and Protocel® passed the toxicity test superbly proving it to be less toxic than an aspirin a day. However, the owners and distributors of Protocel® cannot claim any effectiveness in its use against disease and there are no 'official' studies or trials that have been done on it because of the cancer industry's suppression efforts. At least Jim Sheridan finally saw his unique cancer treatment come to market, even though it was never officially recognized as such. Sheridan passed away in May of 2001 at the age of 90.

One interesting historical anecdote reported by Sheridan was the following. When he worked at Dow Chemical between 1935 and 1946, he was on friendly terms with the head of the company, who was of course Dr. Willard Dow. At one point, Jim went to Dr. Dow and asked him for $200 to buy mice to run cancer experiments on. Dr. Dow liked Jim and therefore decided to refuse him the money. With the keen insight typical to Dow, he told Sheridan that *if he started down that road, he would be forever in conflict with the medical establishment and the federal government.* Apparently Dr. Dow was already aware of suppression efforts by the medical establishment seventy years ago.

Using Protocel®

Protocel® is very easy to use compared to most alternative cancer treatments. It does not involve taking mountains of supplements, intravenous treatments, juicing, or frequent enemas. (Though coffee enemas or colonics can be a helpful adjunct for some people.) In fact, I have come across quite a lot of full recoveries from cancer patients who simply took approximately one-quarter to one-third teaspoonful of the formula in water four or five times a day, spaced out as evenly as possible, and simply took one or two other supplements along with it. Dietary restrictions with Protocel® are minimal and simply suggest cutting out refined sugar, refined flour and alcohol as much as possible and eating a well-balanced healthy diet otherwise while avoiding most common supplements or concentrated foods.

There are two formulations of the Protocel® formula. One is called "Protocel® Formula 23" and the other is called "Protocel® Formula 50". The Formula 23 seems to work best for certain types of cancer, such as breast, prostate, bladder, kidney, and most primary brain cancers, while the Formula 50 seems to work best for other types of cancer, such as lung, liver, colon, cervical, uterine cancer, and melanoma. *All the people in the case stories presented in this chapter used the Formula 50 for their lung cancer.*

The only difficulty in usage is that multiple doses need to be taken every day, and for best results one of those doses should be in the middle of the night. The reason for this is that keeping a therapeutic level of the formula in one's body at all times is very important for its long-term effectiveness and it is recommended to never go more than 6 hours between any two doses. For instance, a common way to start using Protocel® Formula 50 would be to simply take a quarter teaspoonful in distilled water at 8 am, 2 pm, 8 pm, and then 2 am. Doing this every single day and not missing doses is important. As the person finds out how his or her body is handling the cancer breakdown, they may at some point increase their dose to a third of a teaspoonful or more.

Even though this liquid treatment is easy to use, one issue that should be understood before starting to take Protocel® is that there are many vitamins, minerals, herbs, or concentrated juices that *cannot* be taken along with Protocel®. The major conflict here is that Protocel® is designed to deprive cancer cells of energy, while most supplements work to supply the body's cells with *more* energy in one way or another. In this age of nutritional supplementation, it is difficult for some cancer patients to accept that they cannot take a lot of other nutritional supplements along with this treatment. Some of the common supplements that absolutely *must* be avoided are: vitamin C, vitamin E, CoQ10, selenium, IP6, fish oil, and alpha-lipoic acid. (And this is just a partial list – other supplements, herbs, and treatments to avoid are listed in my book as well.)

Even frequent fresh juices and concentrated green drinks are not recommended along with Protocel®, because these concentrated foods are dense in nutrients and may act more like supplements.

But there *are* some excellent anti-cancer supplements that are known to be compatible with Protocel®. For instance, intravenous Laetrile treatments, B17 tablets, and apricot pits are all compatible with Protocel®. Pure ellagic acid, a natural compound from red raspberries that has been proven to help induce apoptosis (natural cell death) in lung cancer cells, is also compatible. And curcumin is compatible. Preliminary studies on curcumin have shown that it blocks the invasion and metastases of lung cancer cells by activating a tumor suppressor protein called HLJ1. Though I have no cases of lung cancer patients using curcumin along with Protocel® to report on, I know that one woman successfully used Protocel® Formula 50 every 6 hours along with just one high-dose capsule (875 mg from Swanson's) of curcumin once a day to make her deadly glioblastoma multiforme brain tumors shrink in size and completely stop highlighting on scans. Scientific studies have shown curcumin to be effective against glioma brain cancers, lung cancer, prostate cancer, breast cancer, and colon cancer, and possibly other types of cancer as well.

Another herb that has been used very successfully for years along with Protocel® is paw paw. Paw paw is similar to graviola, both are compatible with Protocel® and both have been used successfully for lung cancer. But some people believe there are more acetogenins in paw paw, and Nature's Sunshine has a capsule form with standardized ingredients that many Protocel® users like. It has been observed to work synergistically with Protocel® to cause cancer cells to lyse faster in some cases. Paw paw has also been proven in laboratory studies to disarm multi-drug-resistant (MDR) cancer cells that may have been caused by previous chemotherapy, so for any patients who have already done a lot of chemo, taking paw paw every day can be an excellent adjunct to their treatment program.

But, overall, it is important to keep the number of other supplements taken along with Protocel® to a minimum. Thus, for those people who want to take a *lot* of supplements, herbs, fresh-squeezed juices or green drinks on a daily basis, Protocel® may not be the best choice for them. There are other alternative options that are also powerful which can be used with virtually as many supplements as one wants, and some of those options are also presented in my book. For instance, Cesium High pH Therapy, the Flaxseed Oil and Cottage Cheese approach, Dr. Kelley's Metabolic Enzyme Therapy, essiac tea, the Hoxsey Therapy, and others are also presented in *Outsmart Your Cancer*, and these can be used with virtually as many different supplements, herbs and juices as one wants. They are not very expensive approaches, either.

For those who do want to use Protocel® for their lung cancer, simply taking Protocel® Formula 50, B12, pure ellagic acid, curcumin, paw paw, and vitamin D3 (if one is not out in the sun a lot) would be more than enough as a daily protocol.

Can Protocel® be Taken Along with Conventional Treatment?

Radiation treatments are compatible and have been used successfully along with Protocel®. The biggest danger to be considered when using radiation for lung cancer, however, is possible damage to the heart. Given Cindy's extremely short prognosis in

Case Story #3, the radiation treatments she received in the beginning may have been necessary to give the Protocel® time to work. But every lung cancer patient must be careful and weigh the pros and cons for their particular case when it comes to radiation to the chest area.

On the other hand, chemotherapy is *not* recommended in most cases with Protocel®. In fact, most chemotherapy drugs run the risk of interfering with Protocel®'s ability to break down cancer cells on the cellular level, so best results are obtained when people do not use chemo at the same time. Though these would not be used for lung cancer, anecdotal evidence seems to indicate that the use of estrogen-blocking drugs for women or testosterone-blocking drugs for men may also reduce this approach's effectiveness.

Surgery in most cases, of course, will not interfere with the Protocel® approach, when the patient is young and strong enough to undergo major surgery. However, it is important to follow the surgery immediately with the Protocel® to stop any cancer from growing back. If the cancer has been allowed to recur, then previous surgery (such as when a large part of the lung has been removed) can sometimes compromise the person's ability to effectively cough up lysed material that needs to come out.

Some Personal Observations and Tips

One thing that has not yet been proven by studies, but is an observation of my own, is that Protocel® appears to work faster on fast-growing cancers and slower on slow-growing cancers. I believe this is because fast-growing cancers have a higher rate or amount of anaerobic cell respiration than slow-growing cancers do. This concept is supported by various sources of scientific research. For example, more than two decades ago, Dr. Dean Burk, who was head of the cytochemistry department of the National Cancer Institute, conducted a series of experiments where the fermentation (glycolysis) rates of various cancers that grew at different speeds were measured. Dr. Burk and his colleague, Mark Woods, showed that the cancers with the fastest growth rates also had the highest fermentation rates and the cancers with slower growth rates had lower fermentation rates. Later studies by Pietro Gullino at the NCI and Silvio Fiala, a biochemist from the University of Southern California, are reported to have confirmed Dr. Burk's findings. Since the anaerobic cell respiration of cancer cells (which can be referred to either as glycolysis or the fermentation of glucose) is what Protocel® targets and blocks, it makes sense that those fast-growing cells which rely most heavily on glycolysis for their energy would succumb and break down the fastest.

It has also been my observation that annual flu shots interfere with peoples' recoveries on Protocel®. Again, this has not been proven in studies, but I've observed a number of cancer patients who were doing well and were seeing their cancer go away on this formula, then they got a flu shot and experienced their tumors immediately growing again. It is unknown as to whether the mercury, formaldehyde, squalene, or other toxic chemicals in the flu vaccines directly interfere with the formula, or whether the vaccines just cause problems by negatively impacting the patient's immune system. At any rate, I would say: *Avoid All Flu Shots for Best Results With This Approach.*

As already stated, because of the way that Protocel® breaks down cancer cells, people using this liquid formula for lung cancer may experience a certain amount of coughing up of mucousy material. This is simply the broken-down cancer cells or 'lysed material' that the body is processing out. Thus, patients must be able to cough and should also try to drink a lot of water every day to keep their mucous or lymph fluid from becoming too thick.

Though no one likes to think of cancer metastasizing to the brain, lung cancer is one type of cancer that can readily go to the brain. Radiation is often able to reduce tumors in the brain but is rarely curative in the long-term, and chemotherapy drugs are largely ineffective on cancer of any type in the brain. Fortunately, Protocel® works exceedingly well on all types of cancer in the brain, including metastases from lung cancer.

Also already mentioned, when people have used chemotherapy extensively for their cancer before starting Protocel®, they may want to take paw paw along with it to help disarm any possible multi-drug-resistant cancer cells that may have developed.

Another tip is that pneumonia can sometimes highlight on PET scans in a way that may look like cancer. Since lung cancer patients may have compromised lung functioning while they are trying to recover, they are often susceptible to complications such as pneumonia. It is always a good idea to speak directly to one's doctor about whether a highlighting area of the lung on a PET scan is new cancer growth or whether it could possibly be pneumonia instead, which might be treatable with antibiotics.

Are the Rich and Famous with Cancer Better Off?

After reading the case stories in this chapter, it is obvious that Protocel® is an inexpensive approach that most people can afford. But that doesn't mean it is not a good choice for wealthy cancer patients as well. In fact, one misunderstanding is that those with more money, such as the rich and famous, have a better chance of recovering from their cancer because they can afford the 'best possible treatments'.

If they choose to use their money for alternative treatment, this may be true. However, I think the rich and famous are often the ones who are *least* likely to choose alternative medicine when they have cancer. I am guessing this is because they think their money will buy them the very best doctors and treatments in mainstream medicine and that this will give them the very best chance for beating their illness. Unfortunately, top doctors and clinics offering conventional medicine have little to offer that is any different from what lower-ranked conventional doctors or clinics can offer.

The real question is *not* how expensive a treatment is, but whether the treatment has a good chance of working or not. It is my belief that the rich and famous may in fact be *worse* off in their chances for recovery because they don't understand the real issue, which is that *more money cannot buy better cancer treatments within the conventional medical system.*

The bottom line is that what we need is not more money to find 'a cure', but honesty in the cancer industry and an open policy towards evaluating all possible treatments with equal attention. And let's start with clinical trials on those approaches that have already been proven to work by thousands of people who have used them! Until that happens, Protocel® can be ordered as a dietary supplement by cancer patients who are looking for an alternative option to the toxic and largely ineffective treatments conventional medicine has to offer.

Selected Physical/Environmental Interventions: For Treating Lung Cancer and Preventing Recurrence

This chapter will explain how to carry out some of the physical and environmental interventions mentioned throughout the book. These interventions were used both during and following the author's experience with cancer. Thus, they may relate specifically to lung cancer or to good health to prevent a recurrence of cancer. Research related to the value of each will also be presented. The interventions are based upon current scientific data and are safe for most. However, I advise you to consult your primary care physician or practitioner before starting any regime whether exercise or a new diet.

Physical

The interventions included under this heading are smoking cessation, physical exercises and nutrition (maintaining alkalinity, avoiding genetically modified foods and other contaminants).

Smoking Cessation

Smoking is the number one leading cause of preventable deaths in the US. In 1994 there were over 419,000 tobacco related deaths (Gunby). In addition, over 90% of all cases of lung cancer are a result of primary or secondary smoking. Thus, for health reasons, smoking cessation is important. There are three steps to the process of smoking cessation and all are important. These include preparation, the actual quitting, and the maintance of being smoke free.

Preparing to Quit

a) Review your smoking history using an assessment guide such as that found at the end of this section.

b) Determine a date to quit and the amount of nicotine to reduce during the process.

c) Keep a smoking diary.

d) Learn and/or begin relaxation techniques such as those identified in another section of this chapter.

e) Select and start an exercise program (see section on exercise in this chapter). It is best to be exercising 2 or 3 months before quitting.

f) Learn and/or use imagery (discussed in Chapter 10). For example, imagine a place where you usually smoke and then replace this with an image of being in the same place but drinking a glass of water or chewing gum.

g) Write a self-contract for quitting smoking. In the contract include rewards for every 5 to 7 days of success or penalties for failure, finding a support partner, identifying negative and positive thoughts with examples such as "I am more nervous since I quit smoking" to be replaced with "I am aware of a changed mood since I quit smoking and I am replacing this with relaxation and imagery. These make me feel better and healthier".

h) Establish a plan to visit family and friends on your first smoke-free day when your confidence may be low.

i) Determine your high-risk situations and decide ways to prevent a relapse in these situations such as social situations, emotional upset, work frustration, relaxation after eating, or interpersonal conflict.

j) Identify your personal reasons for quitting such as "reducing your risk of lung cancer, and increasing your endurance and productivity". A strong desire is usually required to quit smoking.

k) Decide the best way for you to quit. Choices may include:

1) quit abruptly (cold turkey).

2) Use a slow process of nicotine replacement therapy (NRT) such as gradually withdraw by buying a lower tar and nicotine brand of cigarettes each week for three weeks and prevent a sudden fall of nicotine in the blood supply. This reduces the craving and symptoms of withdrawal. A similar approach is to use nicotine gum, patches, lozenges, or inhalers.

3) Another self-help approach (focused or rapid approach) should only be attempted under supervision if you have heart disease or diabetes. For this unpleasant experience, have the following: cigarettes and matches, wastebasket, candles and holder, pen or pencil and paper to record your responses. Select a place for the experience and arrange the supplies. Have the wastebasket handy in case of vomiting. Light a candle and then light a cigarette from the flames and take a puff every 6 seconds. Upon finishing one cigarette immediately light and puff on another. Continue until you are nauseated, you have smoked three cigarettes or more, and further smoking is impossible because of the unpleasant response. Record the response and repeat the process. Unpleasant responses to record may include: hot lips, mouth and/or tongue, burning throat, burning lungs, pounding heart, dizziness, tingling hands and legs, watery eyes, flushed face, nausea and/or headache.

4) Some other approaches to smoking cessation require outside assistance. One approach is acupuncture combined with a citrate compound. Go for a single acupuncture session and an oral administration of a citrate compound that causes the urine to become alkaline and retain urinary excretion of nicotine. This prevents a sudden fall in nicotine blood levels thereby reducing the craving for nicotine and decreases the withdrawal symptoms. Dossey and Keegan (2008) say this is a rapid

way to quit. Another is the use of Wellbutrin SR (an antide-pressant) that is taken over an extended period of time under medical supervision. This is a prescribed medication. Another approach used successfully by some people is the Nicotrol Inhaler that gives nicotine when inhaled and is based upon a slow reduction in nicotine levels similar in principle to the use of citrate compound.

l) Learn about herbs and vitamins that may be useful during quitting. Some have been advocated to correct possible smoke-related deficiencies and damage while working to quit the habit. Different authorities advocate different antioxidants and supplements to correct deficiencies and damage to the lungs and two follow. Dr. Emanuel Opara (2001) recommends the following: vitamin C 500 to 2000 mg/da and vitamin E (alpha-tocopherol) 400 to 800 iu day (but doses up to 3,200 iu per day have been reported to be safe). He says a combination of these antioxidants work better than one alone and using vitamin C 500 to 1500 mg/da and vitamin E 400 to 800 iu/da is suggested. He also suggests fish oil that has a high content of fat-soluble antioxidants as prevention for smoking-related diseases. Glutathione, a cellular antioxidant useful for the normal functioning of the lungs, was also recommended in the form of N-Acetyl cysteine (NAC) 600 mg/da. He also recommended green tea for its antioxidant and anti-smoking damage properties. Also recommended were: lipoic acid at 100 mg/da, taurine at 1.5 gm/da, coenzyme Q 10 at 90 mg/da, selenium at 200 mcg/da, garlic, ginkgo biliba, and red wine polyphenola.

Dr. Ronald Hoffman (2011) suggested the following for smoking cessation: vitamin C 1000 mg three times a day; vitamin A up to 10,000 iu daily to heal the mucous membrane; CoQ10 50 mg/twice daily to protect the cardio pulmonary system; lipoic Acid 300 mg twice daily, and zinc

30 mg/da for healing of mucous membrane.

Balch & Balch (1997) also suggested supplements for smoking cessation. They advocated vitamin C 5,000 to 20,000 mg daily to protect against cell damage and to replenish depletions in the body due to smoking. Vitamin B complex 100 mg daily in sublingual form repair damage to the cellular system that is often damaged by smoking. Vitamin B12 1000 mg twice daily in lozenge or sublingual form may improve liver functioning and increase energy. Folic acid 400 mg daily for the red blood cells and for cell division and replication. Use vitamin E (an important antioxidant) starting with 200 iu daily and increasing by 200 iu monthly until you reach 800 iu; if tolerated that will protect cells and organs from the harmful effects of smoking. Coenzyme Q10 200 mg twice daily protects the heart and acts as an antioxidant to protect cells and the lungs and aids oxygen flow to the brain. Oxy-5000 Forte from American Biologicals, two tablets 3 times a day destroys free radicals produced by smoking and is thus a powerful antioxidant. Other important herbs and vitamins for the smoker who is quitting are in their book.

m) Identify a partner to quit with you, if possible.

Quitting

Quitting involves implementing your plan developed during the planning phase. Specific items follow.

a) Implement your smoking cessation plan.
b) Review the self-contract and implement the actions, thoughts, and reward system established.
c) Combine a cleansing program with your smoking cessation intervention. This should include frequent bathing to remove toxins, and frequent drinking water to flush your system, which will facilitate the quitting

process.

d) The cleansing program should also include the environment. Replace the filters in your air condition and/or heating system, clean your carpets, drapes, clothing and car interior to remove all odors of smoking.

e) Implement or continue your exercise and relaxation programs planned to increase energy, reduce the possibility of weight gain, and decrease stress. Specifics of exercise and relaxation will be discussed later in this chapter.

f) Use helpful positive affirmations, and imagery. Specific helpful affirmations might include "I am happy to be a non-smoker"; "I am now healthy and happy"; "My lungs are now clear and I can breathe easily". You might think of other positive affirmations that will help you in the process. Affirmations and imagery will be discussed in the next chapter on mental and spiritual interventions.

g) Obtain adequate rest and nutrition to facilitate smoking cessation and prevent weight gain. Weight gain has been reported as a result of smoking cessation and is usually due to overeating and the lack of exercise. The exercise program identified as part of your contract will help.

h) Change your daily routine: 1) On a sheet of paper record the usual events or situations that trigger your smoking such as upon rising in the morning, reading the newspaper, or while relaxing after meals. 2) Next to these events identify new habits to replace the old ones. For example, if coffee triggers smoking, replace it with tea. Likewise, if you frequently light cigarettes keep gum nearby and reach for it instead. Visualizing your new habits will also help.

Smoking Assessment Directions: Are you addicted to cigarettes, or is your smoking just a habit. Answer the following questions to learn more about your smoking behavior.

How soon after you wake up do you smoke your first cigarette?

a. after 30 minutes (0)
b. within 30 minutes (1)

Is it difficult to refrain from smoking in places where it is forbidden such as the library, theatre, or doctor's office?

yes (1)
no (0)

Which of all of the cigarettes you smoke in a day is the most satisfying one?

any other than the first one in the morning (0)
the first one in the morning (1)

How many cigarettes a day do you smoke?
1–15 (0)
16–25 (1)
20 or more (2)

Do you smoke more during the morning than the rest of the day?

yes (1)
no (0)

Do you smoke when you are so ill that you are in bed most of the day?

yes (1)
no (0)

Does the brand you smoke have a low, medium, or high nicotine content?

low (0.9 mg or less) (0)
medium (1.0–1.2 mg) (1)
high (1.3 mg or more) (2)

How often do you inhale the smoke from your cigarette?

a. never (0)
b. sometimes (1)
c. always (2)

Evaluation: To get your score, add the points (found in parentheses) beside each of your responses. The questions are scored so that the higher points are given for answers that reflect a higher level of addiction to cigarettes. A total score of 8 or better reflects a significant probability of nicotine dependence.

Smoking behaviors are typically a complex combination of nicotine dependence and habituation. Nicotine is a highly addictive drug and is considered by some physicians to be more addictive than alcohol or cocaine. Smoking occurs mostly due to automatic behaviors in response to feelings or to situations that are often stressful.

Source: US Department of Health and Human Services, (1986) *Clinical Opportunities for Smoking Interventions.* National Heart, Lung, and Blood Institute, No. 86-2178, August

Smoking Knowledge Directions: Answer each of the following statements with a yes or no.

Yes No
1. I know the effects of smoking on health.
2. I know techniques that facilitate smoking cessation.
3. I know herbs and vitamins that facilitate smoking

cessation.

4. I know the usefulness of meditation and visualization on smoking cessation.

Evaluation: If you answered no to any of the above, you have a knowledge deficit regarding smoking. If you wish to increase your knowledge or quit smoking, techniques for doing this were presented earlier. You are making a positive step toward improving your health.

A CD on smoking cessation is available for sale with additional information on my website: www.holistichealth show.com. It includes an interview with Dr. Scott McIntosh from the University of Rochester who discusses internet resources useful for those quitting smoking.

Research on Smoking Cessation

Research on Smoking Cessation Methods According to the Office of Smoking and Health of the Department of Health and Human Services (1989) concludes tobacco use is responsible for one out of every six deaths and is the most preventable cause of death and disability in the US. It is a major risk factor for diseases of the heart and blood vessels, chronic bronchitis and emphysema, a variety of cancers, and respiratory infections (Office of Smoking and Health, 1989). Passive smoking in non-smokers causes lung cancer in adults and respiratory infections in children. It is also responsible for limitation of activities in individuals with chronic bronchitis, emphysema, and lung cancer. In 1983 to 1987 it accounted for 3% of all activity limitation and was the main cause of activity limitation in 4 out of every 1000 (LaPlant et al, 1988). So how effective are smoking cessation techniques? It was reported (CDC, 1992) that in 1990 there were approximately 46 million adults in the United States who continued to smoke, but there were also more than 44 million people who had quit smoking.

Schwartz (1991) found that self-help techniques such as outlined in this section are cost effective and that hypnosis and acupuncture as quitting techniques are not warranted by the quit rates. Fiore (1990) also concludes that self-help methods are successful and said 90% of successful quitters have used a self-help quitting strategy, most by quitting abruptly. These self-help methods might include quitting cold turkey, using quitting manuals, or using non-prescription drugs. On the other hand about 8% use an assisted method such as smoking cessation clinics, hypnosis, acupuncture, or nicotine patches with counseling and those using clinics tend to be heavy smokers. Cohen et al (1989) looked at twelve-month abstinence rates for those who use self-help methods and concluded the rate for smoking cessation ranges from 8% to 25%. The Public Health Service (1987) looked at this rate for those using assisted strategies and concluded they ranged from 20% to 40%.

Other methods that have been used effectively include mass media campaigns and televised self-help clinics combined with social support (Fray, 1987) and physical counseling (US Preventive Service Task Force, 1999). Kottke et al (1988) evaluated 39 controlled studies on smoking cessation in the literature that looked at 108 interventions in medical practice and concluded: 1) for the type of intervention face-to-face interventions were better than all others; 2) for the person quitting both physician and non-physician counselors together were better than either alone; 3) the number of reinforced sessions and duration of reinforcing sessions were related to successful smoking cessation 6 months after the initial intervention; and 4) a team of physicians and non-physicians using multiple intervention modalities used on multiple occasions produced the best outcome; success after 12 months was related to the type of sessions (group and individual better than either alone) as well as the number of interventions used and the number of reinforced sessions.

Exercise

Anti-Aging Exercises

One of the exercise series I use daily to remain healthy is the Anti-aging or Fountain of Youth exercises. These were discussed in the *Ancient Secret of the Fountain of Youth* (Kelder, 1989) and are supposed to reverse the aging process by many years. The exercises are similar to yoga but are intended to correct imbalances in the body's seven energy centers. These should be performed daily and are most effective for individuals over 40 years of age. The individual should start with three repetitions of each rite daily for a week and then increase it by two repetitions a week until he/she reaches 21 repetitions. Thereafter, 21 repetitions should be performed daily. Each rite should be performed immediately after the preceding one. It is possible to miss one day a week but no more. It is also possible to carry out half of the repetitions in the morning and half at night.

Rite 1 consists of standing erect with arms outstretched and horizontal to the floor. Spin your body around from left to right until you become slightly dizzy. It is helpful to focus on an object each time you return to the starting point. Although children can do many repetitions, this becomes more difficult as you become older. Do not go beyond being slightly dizzy and sit afterwards, if needed. As you continue to perform the rites you will be able to increase the number of these until you reach 21 repetitions.

Rite 2 consists of lying flat on the floor with your face up and your arms fully extended along your side. Keep the fingers close together. Raise your head off the floor with your chin tucked against your chest. At the same time lift your legs with knees straight into a straight upward position. If possible, extend the legs further back toward the head but only if the legs are straight. Slowly lower the legs and head to the floor. Relax and repeat. Breathe in deeply as you lift your legs and head and breathe out as you lower them. Note that this is the opposite of most exercises and yoga.

Rite 3 consists of kneeling on the floor with the body erect. Then lower the head forward tucking the chin against the chest. Next throw the head and neck back as far as it will go and at the same time arch your back as far back as it will go. Brace your arms and hands against your thighs for support as you arch backwards. Return to the original position and repeat. Breathe in deeply as you arch and breathe out as you return to the erect position.

Rite 4 consists of sitting on the floor with body erect and with legs straight out in front of you with your feet about 12 inches apart. Place the palms of the hands on the floor beside the buttocks and tuck your chin against the chest. Then drop the head backwards as far as it will go and raise your body so the knees bend while the arms remain straight. The trunk of the body and upper legs will be elevated and horizontal to the floor. At the same time the arms and lower legs will be perpendicular to the floor. Tense every muscle and return to the original position. Relax as you return and rest before repeating. Breathe in deeply as you raise the body and breathe out as you lower it.

Rite 5 starts with your body face down toward the floor supported by the hands with palms down against the floor and the toes in a flexible position. The toes and feet should be about 2 feet apart. At the start of the rite the arms will be perpendicular to the floor with the spine arched. Throw the head back as far as possible and bend at the hips bringing the body up into an inverted V position, Concurrently tuck the chin against the chest. Return to the original position. Breathe in deeply as you raise the body and exhale as you lower it.

Modified from: Kelder, Peter (1989) *Ancient Secret of the Fountain of Youth*. Gig Harbor, WA: Harbor Press, Inc.

Anti-Aging Exercise Research

Although there is no research on the effects of this series of rites on a daily basis, the book quotes practitioners as having more energy, a better memory, looking and feeling younger, loosing fat and flab, and curing a variety of conditions from arthritis to sinus problems to pain. I have used these rites for many years and am always told I look 15 or more years younger, rarely have aches and pains, have no chronic health problems, and have no difficulty walking 5 to 7 miles a day. I am 79 years of age. It is difficult to tell how much of this good health is a result of genetics or of other daily practices such as positive mental affirmations, meditation, and prayer. However, I believe these are beneficial to everyone over 40. In addition, the exercises are similar to yoga and there is much research on the value of that practice.

Other exercises:

Living in a 3-story house I am up and down stairs several times a day. I also walk from 2 to 4 miles a day on the beach usually around 7 am. I also do a few exercises to maintain strength in my arms and back by lifting 2-pound weights and also using a 2-string chest pull. I maintain my abdomen by using the abdomen roller in the morning and my flexibility using the anti-aging exercises.

Some calories burned by selected exercises in calories burned/minute are:

Walking–brisk (245/30): Jogging–10 minute mile (348/30); Bicycling (206/30);
Aerobic dance or jazzercise (276/30); Swimming (290/30); Dancing (105/30);
Tennis (222/30) and Weight lifting (200/30).

You can burn 150 calories a day with the following physical activities: 30 minute non-brisk walk; 15 minute run; or washing and waxing your car for 45 minutes according to the Surgeon General's Report on physical activity. They further say 30 minutes of moderate activity daily will reduce the risk of coronary heard disease, type 2 diabetes, hypertension, and colon cancer and will improve your physical and mental health (US Department of Health and Human Services, 1996).

Precautions

Any exercise program should be preceded by a medical evaluation. Factors such as physical condition, chronic illness, blood pressure, family history, and medications may alter exercise patterns. Individuals can be classified as having: 1) no risk factors for exercise; or 2) having risk factors and/or disease. Some conditions that may preclude participating in conditioning exercise programs are a recent history of myocardial infarction, recent pulmonary embolism, congestive heart failure, acute infections, heart block (second and third degree), aortic aneurysm, acute myocarditis, severe valvular disease, and uncontrolled arrhythmia.

Warm-Up and Cool-Down Exercise Phases

Although they do not provide a conditioning effect, warm-up and cool-down periods are important parts of exercise programs. The warm-up phase increases blood flow and stretches postural muscles and thereby prepares the body for sustained activities. This prevents a sudden increase in workload on the heart, the circulatory system, and the muscles and joints.

These should be preformed for 5 or 10 minutes until your heart rate slowly reaches a safe range of pulse or heartbeats per minute. The following types of warm up are suggested: 1) rhythmic movements such as knee bends or walking with hands clasped behind your head while twisting side to side (rotation of the trunk). 2) Stretching exercises such as touching toes, raising hands over head and bending side to side, progressing to knee hugs, straight knee raises, and walking rapidly in a circle.

The cooling down period is equally important to prevent

fainting or a brief loss of consciousness resulting from a sudden decrease in the blood flow to large muscle groups. For 5 or 10 minutes you should: 1) continues to use the large muscle groups such as jogging but at a slower pace; 2) a few minutes of slow walking; and 3) range of motion, stretching, and static muscle contraction and relaxation.

Exercise Pyramid

A physical activity and exercise pyramid was presented by the McKinley Health Center at the University of Illinois in Urbana-Champagne (2000). It describes various exercises, recommended frequency and intensity of each, and the duration of performance. Aerobic exercises, strength training, and flexibility are all incorporated into the pyramid. Level I (the base) of the pyramid include moderate everyday activities (walking stairs instead of using elevators, walking to work, cleaning house, gardening, laundry, dancing, shopping) for at least 30 minutes daily. This fulfills guidelines for physical activity established by the US Surgeon General.

Level II of the pyramid includes aerobic or cardiac activities such as jogging or bicycling, and more vigorous activities (sports and recreational) such as tennis, volleyball, and hiking, step aerobics, cardio machines, and cardio-boxing. It is most beneficial if activities from both categories are included for 30 minutes or more for 3 days a week.

Level III and IV involves flexibility and muscle fitness (muscle strength such as the amount of weights used in bench pressing) activities and muscle endurance (how long you perform the exercise). Flexibility exercises include stretching exercises and should include the full range of motion for muscle groups for 3 to 7 days a week. In addition, the American College of Sports Medicine recommends strength training at least 2 days a week with a day of rest between. Repetitions and number of sets for weight training are identified. They also include high intensity activities and competitive sports at the fourth level. At the top of the pyramid is inactivity. A person who has lived a sedentary life should start with activities from Level I and build slowly from there.

This pyramid has been modified to accommodate individuals with various health conditions. For example, a plan for the individual with arthritis includes 4 levels. The bottom level recommends the following daily: taking extra steps during the day, walking the dog, and parking the car further away and walking. Level II recommends recreational sports and aerobic activities 3 to 5 times weekly. Level III recommends stretching and strengthening exercises and enjoying leisure activities 2 or 3 times weekly. The top level recommends sitting sparingly.

I Research on Exercise

Research shows that regular exercise can help prevent and manage coronary heart disease, hypertension, insulin dependent diabetes, osteoporosis, obesity and mental health problems such as depression and anxiety (Harris et al, 1989). People who are physically active tend to live longer than those who are inactive (Harris et al, 1989; Paffenbarger, 1986) and similar results were found in the Multiple Risk Factor Intervention Trial (Leon, 1987). This was a 7-year follow-up of over 12,000 men and the death rate for those with moderate activity was 70% less than those with low activity. Physical activity increases the quality of life (Katz et al, 1983) and helps the elderly remain independent in physical activities (Katz, 1983). Regular exercise has also been associated with decreased rates of colon cancer (Powell et al, 1989), stroke (Salonen et al, 1982) and reduced back injury (Cady et al, 1979). The Diabetes and Health News website (1999) states that inactivity contributes to 250,000 deaths yearly.

Numerous studies have researched cardiovascular disease and exercise. Salonen (1988), Curfman (1993), Garcia-Palmieri (1982), and Hambrecht (1993) all found a positive relationship. In

1994, Lakka studied over 1400 Finnish men between ages 42 and 60 and found that those who reported more than two hours of exercise weekly had a 60% reduction in their risk of heart disease compared to a group of less active men. Sandvik (1993) found similar results in a group of Norwegian men. Berlin (1990) reviewed studies of heart disease and exercise and found being sedentary almost doubled the risk for developing coronary heart disease. Katz (1983) found the same results. The risk of coronary heart disease from inactivity is only slightly less than from smoking, high blood pressure, and high blood cholesterol. More people are at risk of coronary heart disease from the lack of physical activity than from any other risk factor (PHS, 1990).

Manson (1992) found that physicians who exercised only once a week experienced a decrease of 23% risk of diabetes, and those who exercised 5 or more times a week reduced their risk by 42%. Helmrich (1991) presented similar results. In his study of alumni from the University of Pennsylvania there was a 6% reduction in the risk of diabetes for each 500 calories expended in weekly exercise. Earlier studies also found a lower risk for cancer (Albanese, 1989; Bernstein, 1994) and depression (Ross, 1988; Klein, 1985; and McCann, 1984) in those participating in daily physical activity.

Recent studies continue to find a value in regular physical activity. Courneya (2003) reviewed 47 published articles on cancer survivors and physical activities and concluded that preliminary results suggest that physical exercise in cancer survivors improve their quality of life. Over 50 studies have been reported on the relationship of colorectal cancer and physical activity and many have consistently found that adults who increase their physical activity (intensity, duration, frequency) can reduce their risk of colorectal cancer by 30 to 40% regardless of body mass index and the greatest risk reduction is seen among those most active (Slattery, 2004; IARC Handbooks of Cancer, 2002; Ballard et al, 2006; Lee, 2006; McTiernan, 2006). Twenty-one studies were found on the relationship of lung cancer and physical activity. Most of these find an inverse relationship between lung cancer and physical activity so that the more active individual may have up to a 20% reduction in risk (Lee, 2006; IASRC Handbooks of Cancer, 2006). Many more studies showing the improved quality of life and reduced risk of developing cancer as a result of physical activity can be found on my blog at www.holistichealthshow.com or by a Google search.

Nutrition
Maintaining Alkalinity in the Body
Testing Body Alkalinity
Litmus paper or pH Test Strips are useful for testing alkalinity in the body and can be obtained at http://www.vaxa.com/913.cfm. Remove strip (do not touch yellow end) and insert yellow end into the urine flow. The color change on the yellow portion of the strip can be compared with the chart provided and will indicate where you fall on the acid-alkalinity scale. Most researchers believe it is best to remain somewhat near 7 to 7.5 on this scale although your body will fluctuate over time (see the Healthy Urine Table in the kit).

Maintaining Alkalinity
There are many products on the market to assist in this process. Food and minerals are the natural way to do this. One of the best foods to use is lemon. Squeeze one or two lemons into a glass of water and drink in the morning. I usually add some stevia (the only natural sugar substitute) for sweetening. Minerals are also useful. I prefer Xooma Xtreme 2-0 purchased locally from Xooma Worldwide at www.xoomaworldwide.com for the nearest location to you. I add three X2-0 sachets into a half-gallon of filtered or spring water, shake and let stand for 20 minutes and then drink this water during the day. This provides enough calcium, magnesium and trace minerals to move me toward an

adequate alkalinity level. Measuring out ½ gallon of water daily also assures that I drink an adequate amount of water to avoid dehydration (a common problem among the elderly).

Genetically Modified and Irradiated Foods:

Introduction

Genetically modified refers to foods in which the genetic makeup has been altered by transferring one or more genes from another organism. This is most often seen in plant foods to make them resistant to pests, disease drought, or temperature variations. It also increases the output of the plant, and may increase nutritional value, shelf life, and improve flavor. Unfortunately, many questions about the safety of this process are unanswered and the government does not require labeling so the consumer knows which foods are modified and which are not. Much of the research has been negative and a well-researched article titled *50 Harmful Effects of Genetically Modified Foods* can be found at: http://healthbeyondhype.com/pdf/harmful_effects.pdf.

It has been estimated that more than 70% of food in grocery stores in the United States currently contains genetically modified ingredients. If a store product contains any of the following ingredients on a label they are *likely genetically modified*: corn, corn flour, dextrin, starch, soy, soy sauce, margarine, and tofu.

Irradiated foods are foods in which ionizing radiation splits molecular bonds with high-energy beams and is used on fruit, vegetables, and meat allowing them to sit on shelves much longer than non-irradiated foods. However, there are tremendous health hazards to this practice. For example, the dose of radiation necessary to irradiate meat is fifteen to twenty million times greater than a chest k-ray and produces elevated levels of benzene, formaldehyde, and other cancer-producing compounds in food. Thousands of studies have been carried out ion-irradiated foods and most results have been negative.

Despite the data, the FDA continues to sanction irradiated foods. Although all irradiated food is suppose to be labeled with a symbol (radura) that resembles a flower with a single leaf on each side, within a circle, this is not always done. In addition, restaurants and schools may use irradiated food.

Avoiding GMF and Irradiated Foods

To avoid these products, readers should do the following: 1) Become knowledgeable about genetically engineered foods. 2) Buy organic foods (have a 5 digit number starting with a '9') that are the only foods that are omitted from the genetically engineered foods, grow your own, or buy food at the local farmers market. 3) Encourage your friends and family to buy organic, grow their own, or buy at the farmers market. 4) Use the political process, join computer network groups or use other methods to bring pressure on federal agencies to test and to label genetically engineered foods. Agencies that may be targeted for this purpose include: the Federal Food and Drug Administration; the Environmental Protection Agency; and the United State Dairy Association. Also write letters to your congressmen, to the editor of your local newspapers, or write articles for the newspaper to educate others about these foods. 5) Sign petitions or get in contact with others who are involved with this problem. Some include: a) Mothers for Natural Law, (515) 472-2809 (Iowa) or http://www.safe-food.org. They have good information and a right to know petition regarding GE foods: b) Campaign for Food Safety Minnesota (218) 226-4164 or http://www.organic-consumers.org/ or alliance@mr.net- they have information on factory farming, GE, and citizen actions. c) http://www.biointegrity.org or infr@bio.integrity.org that coordinate broad-based lawsuits against the FDA for failing to label and demand testing of GE foods; and Physicians and Scientists for Responsible Application of Science and Technology at http://www.psrast.org or info@psrast.org Additional resources will be found using a

Google search on the Internet.

The main way to avoid irradiated food is to buy organic as discussed above.

Organizations that work to end irradiation of food are Organic Consumers Association at http://www.organic-consumers.org/irradlink.cfm, the International Institute of Concern for Public Health www.iicph.org, Public Citizen at http://www.citizen.org/cmep and the Cancer Prevention Coalition at www.preventcancer.com

Because of the extensive information presented in the chapter on nutrition, no additional information will be presented here.

Environmental

Some of the environmental interventions discussed in Chapters 2 and 3 that the author used to recover from and/or prevent a recurrence of lung cancer are discussed below. These include radon and asbestos detection and removal, detecting and overcoming sick building syndrome, and maintaining air quality. Some of these may pertain to you and others may not. For example, if you live in a new house, I would not expect to find asbestos but depending upon where you live radon may be a possibility. If either is found it may need to be dealt with.

Asbestos

Asbestos is one of the causal factors for lung cancer and should always be assessed in your home or workplace. It is not always dangerous – only when it is being removed or if it disintegrates and becomes airborne. Removing or encapsulating asbestos is never recommended unless it is damaged but when remodeling a home it is best to obtain an asbestos survey. In single-family homes individuals may remove the asbestos or obtain the services of a state-certified asbestos abatement contractor. For duplexes or larger units professional services are required.

Many asbestos products should be wetted down with water

before removing to prevent airborne particles. The individual removing the asbestos should wear a respirator, disposable coveralls, goggles, disposable gloves, and rubber boots. Once removed, the materials must be disposed of at a site authorized to receive these hazardous materials.

Radon

Radon is a naturally occurring, invisible, odorless, radioactive gas that comes from natural radioactive deposits in soil, rock, and water. Although it is harmless outside a home where it is diluted, it can be harmful when it seeps in and is trapped inside a house. It is one cause of lung cancer that may occur 5 to 25 years following exposure. Radon levels vary by state and information for your state can be found at: http://www.epa.gov/iaq/wherey-oulive.html. Because other factors besides your geographic area are involved in radon exposure it is always best to test for this gas in your home. For example, some granite countertops have been found to be radioactive and to emit radon (Llope, 2008).

Eliminating Radon

The Environmental Protection Agency (EPA) recommends the following: 1) Have a house tested for radon when buying or selling. 2) Ask if radon-resistant materials were used if buying a new house. 3) Have a house repaired if the radon level is 4 Pico Curies per liter or higher. 4) Radon levels less than that still pose a threat but usually can be reduced using one of the methods discussed below.

Ideally it is best to prevent radon from entering the house. Air pressure differences between air in the house and outside drives the gas through cracks in the house floor. Thus: 1) Seal floors to eliminate radon entry. 2) Reduce radon levels before it enters the house by a) using an under floor sump system that collects the radon in an area the size of a bucket and vents it outside; b) improving ventilation under suspended timber floors; and c) positive ventilation systems that increase pressure thereby preventing seepage into the house. 3) Remove radon if it enters the house. Since smokers are more likely to have lung cancer following exposure to radon, quit smoking. It has other positive effects as well (see smoking cessation interventions earlier in this chapter).

The following radon-resistant features can be built into a new house to prevent radon seepage. You may want to discuss these with your builder. 1) The gas-permeable layer is placed beneath the flooring or slab to allow the gas to move freely under the house. Material for this layer may be 4 inches of clean gravel and is used only in homes with basements or on slabs and not in homes with crawl spaces. 2) Next plastic sheeting is placed on top of the gas-permeating layer and under the slab to help prevent seepage from the gas. 3) Seal and caulk all below-grade openings in the foundation and walls. 4) Run a 3 or 4 PVP vent pipe from the gas-permeable layer through the house to the roof in order to safely vent the radon and other gases to the outside. 5) Place an electrical junction box in the attic so that a vent fan can be wiring and installed.

Testing a home for radon can be done by the homeowner or by a qualified radon tester usually a home inspector. There are two types of Radon devices used for testing: These are Passive and Active. Passive devices do not require power to function-they are put in a house for a specific period of time and then sent to the lab for analysis. They are generally inexpensive and are available at http://www.testproducts.com/safecart. Active testing devices require power to function. They provide continuous monitoring and measuring and recording the amount of radon in the home. Homes can be tested for radon using a short or long-term method. The short-term testing uses a device in the home for 2 to 90 days whereas the long-term tests remain in the home for more than 90 days.

If you have granite countertops and other interior products

that emit radon remove them if possible. If not use a good ventilation system and open the windows as often as possible. More
information on dealing with a radon problem can be found at:
http://www.epa.gov/radon/pubs/hmbyguid.html.

Sick Building Syndrome

Sick Building Syndrome is a current problem in the USA and is a
situation in which there are similar symptoms among occupants
in the building linked to the amount of time spent there.
Symptoms may include anxiety, feelings of spaciness, headache,
irritability, inability to concentrate, and mood swings. These
symptoms may relate to: a) inadequate ventilation; b)
construction products and furnishings that emit fumes; c)
chemicals entering the building; d) cigarette smoke; e) molds and
bacteria circulating in heating and cooling systems; f) florescent
lighting; and g) cleaning solutions and other solvents.

Resolving Sick Building Syndrome

You can resolved this problem by: 1) Opening windows often to
air out the house. 2) Leave a window open slightly in your
sleeping rooms, if possible. 3) Place plants that reduce toxic
emissions in strategic places throughout the house. These may
include the Boston fern, chrysanthemum, ficus, corn plant, dwarf
date palm, and English ivy among others (Crinnion, 2000; Plants
as Purifiers, 1994). For additional, useful plants see your local
nursery. 4) Reduce the toxins emitted in the home by eliminating
certain products or replacing the chemicals used with non-toxic
ones. For example, instead of Drano, use a mixture of vinegar,
salt and baking soda to unclog drains; or dissolve 2 tablespoons
of baking soda in 2 cups of hot water and use as a spray instead
of using commercial aerosols that may contain dichlorobenzene,
a chemical that can be toxic to the nervous system, kidneys, and
liver. On her website, Annie Berthold-Bond (2004) identifies
many non-toxic solutions for household chores. 5) Do not allow

cigarette, cigar or pipe smoking in your house. 6) Immediately wipe up water or other spills and regularly inspect bathrooms or other damp places for evidence of mold. If found, either correct the condition or hire a professional to do it. In addition, Clorox works well to remove mold. Other solutions may be found on the Internet.

Mold can cause major health problems if not resolved. For example, Hurricane Isabel moved three feet of water through the first floor of my house and removal of the wallboard and cleaning of the area with bleach by a contractor was necessary to prevent spread of the mold to the living areas on the second and third floors. This occurred in August when it was hot and humid and without electricity for 10 days mold took over quickly. With exposure of the mold as I removed stored items to the trash pile, I developed allergies that returned seasonally for several years after. 7) Be selective when buying furnishings for you home as many give off fumes that are toxic.

Indoor Air Quality

According to the Environmental Protection Agency the air inside US homes may be any where from 2 to 100 times more polluted than outdoor air and newer homes may have poorer quality air than older ones because they are better insulated to preserve energy. Thus, it is important to maintain air quality within the home to maintain health and prevent recurrence of lung cancer or other diseases.

Maintaining Air Quality

Some things you can do to maintain a clean air supply include: 1) Avoid recontamination by using the correct vacuum. It is best to use a bagless vacuum with a HEPA type filter to prevent dust from escaping back into the air. 2) Periodic servicing of heating system: If you have a forced-air heating system have ducts periodically cleaned and sealed internally. Have the ductwork sealed with Aeroseal that eliminates air leaking from the ductwork behind the drywall and plaster. This will reduce energy bills, and make heat more evenly distributed. Sealing the ductwork reduces dust and dirt that is forced through the return line and makes the air quality better. 3) Use a good quality air filter on your furnace: Upgrading from the cheap spun glass filters to a pleated one that will catch smaller particles improves the quality of the air. Change these regularly. I buy mine at Home Depot for around $18 and change them every 3 months. 4) Install an indoor air purifier. This will filter small particles from the air and make it easier to breathe. 5) Do not allow smoking in your home. 6) Maintain comfortable heating/cooling: Check your home daily and adjust temperatures as needed to provide comfort. 7) Circulate fresh air: Open windows daily, if possible, to eliminate stale air and obtain fresh air. 8) Maintain comfortable humidity: Adjust the humidity as necessary in homes with humidifiers or dehumidifiers. It is possible to add humidifiers to forced-air furnaces to put moisture in the dry air. They can be set for different levels of humidity. I had one added to my older furnace and set it at about 40, which is comfortable. It is serviced annually at the same time as my furnace or air conditioning to make sure the water line is working and there is no mold or other problems. 9) Other quality controls: Other factors that affect air quality such as radon, and asbestos were discussed earlier. In addition, carbon dioxide monitors should be installed throughout the house and checked regularly, replacing batteries when necessary. I change mine each New Year's because it is easier to remember on a specific date. 10) Negative ions for health. You may want to use a negative ion machine to improve air quality and this is discussed next.

Negative Ion Machine

Electrical charges in air that are positive or negative and are necessary for survival are called ions. In nature these are about equally distributed but may shift by geographical location or circumstances. For example, freeway traffic or forced air and air conditioning may reduce the negative ions in air. On the other hand living in the country or near the ocean may increase these ions. Negative ions tend to be exhilarating and increase our sense of well-being.

I have used a negative ion machine periodically since 1992. I use it during the night as I sleep and it makes me feel refreshed and relaxed in the morning. If you find this too exhilarating at night affecting your quality of sleep use it during the day.

The following specifications are based upon my Ion Fountain: Ion Density: variable depending upon output setting from 340,000 ions per CC/Sec at 1 meter with collection panel attached and 540,000 ions per CC/Sec at 1 meter without Collector Panel attached. Power: 110-120 volts AC the standard household current. Ozone-less than 2 parts per billion. Dimensions are 5 3/8 x 4¼ x 2 3/8. The Collector panel is 8 by 8 inches. Weight: 3 pounds. Can be used in a room 12 by 12.

Instructions: 1) Keep the ion fountain collector toward the center of the room at least 3 to 5 feet off the ground and away from grounded electrical appliances such as toasters, telephones and large metal objects (will ground out or neutralize the ion effect). 2) If placed on a desk make sure there is nothing in front of it to obstruct the flow of ions from the emitting surface. 3) Snap the ion fountain to the collector panel. 4) Adjust the output as needed. It is on high when sent from the factory but can be adjusted by turning the output adjustment counterclockwise to lower and clockwise to raise the output. 4) Move the setting to low for sleeping, and to high for a highly polluted or smoky area. 5) For optimum effectiveness place the fountain 2 to 5 feet from yourself.

Research on Negative Ions:
O'Brian (2004) reported on research at the University of

Pennsylvania Graduate Hospital that found 63% of hundreds of patients suffering from hay fever and bronchial asthma administered negative ions experienced partial to total relief. He also reported on several studies that demonstrated the effectiveness of negative ions in the treatment of pain. It is believed that ions act on oxygen absorption. Negative ions in the bloodstream accelerate delivery of oxygen to cells and tissues causing euphoria, whereas positive ions slow down this process producing symptoms similar to oxygen deprivation. Researchers also believe negative ions may stimulate processes in the body that produce resistance to disease. Palti et al (1966) found children with respiratory problems recovered faster, were less prone to relapse and did not cry as much when negative ions were added to the air compared to those who did not receive this intervention. Soyka (1991) reported on a study among victims of asthma, bronchitis, and hay fever. The sample was randomly selected from a list of people who had purchased a negative ion air purifier. Through interviews, they found that 18 of 24 asthmatics, 13 of 17 bronchitis sufferers, 11 of 12 hay fever victims and 6 of 10 sufferers from nasal catarrh, reported that the product had noticeable improved their condition. Some reported that it cured their condition.

Cramer (1996) reports that Brazilian Hospitals commonly use ionizing machines for treating breathing problems. They followed a sample of 36 children with asthmatic allergies and all had consistent and in some cases crippling problems before taking negative ion therapy. During the treatment only one suffered an allergy attack and afterward all were reported cured and no longer suffered problems if they used occasional negative ion therapy.

Summary

This chapter explained how to carry out some of the supplemental physical and environmental interventions useful for treating and preventing lung cancer and for maintaining good health.

Parts of this chapter were reproduced and modified from Helvie, C. (2007) Healthy Holistic Aging, Minneapolis, Minnesota: Syren Books with permission.

Chapter 10

Selected Mental/Spiritual Interventions: For Treating Lung Cancer and Preventing Recurrence

Introduction

Mental and spiritual interventions are an important part of cancer treatment and the prevention of recurrence. This chapter will look at interventions mentioned throughout the book and put them within a framework of stress reduction.

Stress occurs in the lives of all people and, if unchecked, can have major social and health consequences. Techniques can be learned that will eliminate/reduce stress in one's life to avoid these effects. The mental and spiritual interventions are presented here under the stress reduction framework to reinforce a holistic approach to care. Some physical aspects of stress reduction are included to show a holistic approach even though physical interventions were presented in the last chapter. For clarity physical, mental and spiritual aspects of stress reduction are presented separately but a holistic approach using interventions from each category is most effective.

Physical Interventions of Stress Reduction
Diet

Nutrition is one of the first physical-chemical factors to consider when developing a plan to reduce or eliminate stress. Edgar Cayce recommended the Alkaline-based diet to prevent illnesses and this also works well to reduce stress. He identified foods that produce acidity and alkalinity in the body and recommended eating 80% alkaline producing foods and 20% acid producing foods. Some acid producing foods include meat, grains, and sweets and some foods that are alkaline producing include fruit, vegetables, and milk products. He also recommended foods and food combinations that should be avoided such as citrus fruits and cereals at the same meal. You can test for the acid-alkalinity balance in your body using litmus paper discussed in Chapter 9. A table and discussion of this diet can be found in McGarey, W (1989) and additional information was presented in Chapter 9.

When the body becomes too acidic you may experience gastric reflex that further aggravates stress symptoms. Conversely, stress turns the body balance acidic. A natural solution to resolving acid reflux is orange peel containing d-limonene, a product I have used for acid reflux caused by a hiatal hernia. It was very effective and is called Heartburn Free made by Enzymatic Therapy at Enzymatic Therapy, Inc, Green Bay, Wisconsin 54311, at 1-800-783-2286 www.enzy.com. It contains 1,000 mg of orange peel extract standardized to contain a minimum of 98.5% d-limonene. You take one capsule every other day for 20 days and they guarantee that you will be free of acid reflux for 6 months. I also drink aloe vera to soothe the GI Tract.

Chemicals

Avoid chemicals such as smoking and alcohol. If you are a smoker please obtain my smoking cessation ebook and CD that uses a holistic natural approach to smoking cessation.

Activities

Some physical activities you can use to reduce or eliminate stress include:

1) Walk around the block or count to 10 before responding to others in tense situations.
   Physical exercise releases endorphins that elevates mood after 30 minutes and increases oxygen to the brain.
2) Obtain adequate sleep and rest.

Mental Activities
Relaxation

One of the first mental exercises that can be used to reduce stress is relaxation.

There are several variations of relaxation exercises and some of these are presented below. These range from simple head and neck exercises to those that relax the whole body. Using the mind these exercises quiet the body and allow it to rebuild its energy reserve.

Brief Relaxation 1

This is carried out 3 times a day for 5 minutes. 1) Begin by sitting comfortably in a chair and closing your eyes. 2) Concentrate on remembering the most peaceful setting you have been in – it might be a mountain setting, a stream running through a meadow or the sun setting on a lake. 3) With each breath you take think relax, relax. 4) With practice your problems and worries will float away.

Brief Relaxation 2

This is carried out 3 times a day. 1) Close your eyes. 2) Inhale deeply through the nose, hold, and then exhale through the mouth. 3) While exhaling mentally say "one" or "peace". 4) Repeat 5 times.

Brief Relaxation 3

1) Close your eyes. 2) Breath in deeply through the left nostril and exhale through the right (you will need to hold one nostril with your finger). 3) Breathe in through the right nostril and exhale through the left. 4) Breath in through the nose (both nostrils) and exhale through the mouth. Repeat 3 times.

Progressive Relaxation

This method relaxes the 15 to 20 major muscle groups from your feet to your head and reduces stress, headaches, anxiety, and insomnia, and lowers elevated blood pressure. 1) Sit or lie in a comfortable position. Loosen clothing, if necessary. 2) Close your eyes. 3) Concentrate on your breathing. Be aware of breathing in and out. Say "in" and "out" with your breath if it is not distracting. 4) When you are calm begin instructing your muscle groups to relax. Begin by thinking "feet relax, feet relax". Then "calves relax, calves relax", "legs relax, legs relax". Continue with muscle groups until you finish the neck and head. 5) After you complete the relaxation exercises, again focus on your breathing. Do some deep breathing as identified above under brief relaxation exercises. 6) Now you are ready to sit up or stand up and you should feel relaxed.

A variation of this technique is the Progressive Muscle Relaxation and involves tensing and relaxing each muscle group. These exercises are usually carried out once daily. 1) You tense each muscle hard for 7 to 10 seconds but do not strain. You may visualize the muscle group you are tensing. 2) Release the tension abruptly and relax the muscle group for 15 to 20 seconds letting them go completely limp. 3) You may repeat the phrase "I am relaxed" as you relax the muscle. 4) Repeat the tensing and relaxing once on each muscle group.

Research on Relaxation

Research on relaxation exercises has shown them to be effective. In 1988, O'Leary et al studied the effect of relaxation exercises, cognitive pain management, and goal setting on arthritis. The control group received information on arthritis self-management and the experimental group received relaxation exercises and the information. Results showed that the treatment group was less depressed and stressed, slept longer and were better able to cope with their arthritis. In another study by Kohen and Wynne (1997) relaxation, imagery, storytelling and hypnosis were used in a preschool program for children and parents. Symptom severity scores and physician visits for asthma were both significantly reduced in the treatment group.

Several studies have shown that relaxation is effective in reducing the frequency of seizures in epileptic patients. One of the first studies of progressive relaxation use with individuals with seizures studied 8 poorly controlled epileptics. Four of the subjects had progressive relaxation training (PRT) whereas the other four had a fake training program and later PRT. The fake treatment had no effect but the PRT resulted in a 30% reduction in seizures of both groups (Rousseau et al, 1985). In another study of 24 subjects, PRT reduced seizures by 29% compared to a control group that practiced quiet sitting in which the seizure frequency reduced only 3% (Puskarich et al, 1992). Another research group found similar results (Whitman et al, 1990). In another study, Dahl et al (1987) divided 18 epileptic adults into three groups. Group one learned to relax their muscles, identify high-risk situations and apply the learned relaxation techniques to them. The second group received supportive therapy and the third group received no interventions but was asked to record the number of seizures they experienced. Initially, the first group showed a significant decrease in the frequency of seizures. However, in part two of the study, groups two and three were also taught relaxation techniques and after that their seizures decreased significantly. In a second study by Dahl et al (1985) 18 children with severe seizure disorders were assigned to one of three groups: behavioral and relaxation training, no treatment, or attention only. In the ten-week and one-year follow-ups only the relaxation group showed a reduction on a seizure index that measured both the frequency and intensity of the seizures.

In a study on the influence of relaxation on depression, anxiety and mood, Bridge (1988) studied 154 breast cancer patients receiving radiation. They were randomly assigned to one of three groups: progressive muscle relaxation and deep breathing; relaxation and deep breathing with pleasant imagery;

and a control group in which subjects were encouraged to talk about themselves. Before the study all subjects had similar scores on self-rating tools for mood, depression and anxiety. Six weeks after the study began, the first two groups had significantly better mood scores (subjects in the second group had the best), and mood scores were worse in the control group. Depression and anxiety scores were not significantly different in the three groups.

Another research, Holden-Lund (1988) randomly assigned 24 patients scheduled for gallbladder removal to one of two groups. Interventions started the day before surgery. Group one observed 20 minutes of quiet time daily for 5 days and group two watched a 20 minute video on relaxation and guided imagery for 20 minutes daily over the five days. Subjects in group two showed less anxiety following surgery than group one (the control group).

In several studies relaxation has been shown to be effective in pain reduction. Stuckey (1986) found relaxation training was more effective in reducing chronic low back pain than placebos or EMG biofeedback. In another study on pain following spinal surgery, Lawlis (1985) divided 100 patients into two matched groups. Group one received 1 hour of relaxation instructions on the night before surgery, whereas the control group who had the same surgery had no instructions in relaxation. The group receiving relaxation instructions had shorter hospital stays, complained less to nurses, and used less pain medication following surgery.

Another researcher, Kiecolt-Glasser et al (1985) studied the effect of relaxation on the immune system of 45 elderly individuals in an independent living facility. Subjects were divided into three groups: group one received relaxation training three times a week; group two received social contact three times a week; and group three received no planned contact. After a month, group one showed a significant increase in natural killer cell activity, the subjects reported feeling more relaxed and the antibody levels of the herpes virus had dropped. There was no significant change in groups two and three.

In a recent Internet article from the University of Maryland Medical Center (2010) the author states there are over 3,000 articles showing the health effects of relaxation. A search on Google should identify many of these.

Visualization

Visualization (creative imagery) involves using the natural thought processes to obtain a desired outcome. This may be to invoke healing through the body-mind-emotion triad. One exercise that can be practiced three times a day for 10 to 15 minutes follows. After closing your eyes: 1) imagine the illness or stress you are experiencing and visualize it any way you prefer. (You may see the cancer cells as black blobs in your arteries, a headache as marbles rattling around in your head, and viruses as jelly in the arteries.) 2) Picture treatment in your mind and see it eliminating the attackers or strengthening the body. For example, treatment my be visualized as increasing the number of knights on horseback in the arteries that will attack, kill and carry the cancer cells away, or the treatment may be visualized as white cells that eat the jelly and clean the arteries. It may be visualized as pushing the marbles out of the head by way of the nose or mouth, or it may be visualized as receiving healing from God or some other higher being as he lays his hands on you. When I was diagnosed with lung cancer I visualized the white cells as knights on horseback going through my body and attacking and carrying away the cancer cells. When Rue McClanahan from *The Golden Girls* was diagnosed with breast cancer she surrounded herself with angels and prayed to them. She also visualized spaceships that she sent out to obliterate the cancer cells (Campbell, 2004).

Treatment may also be imagined as a cool throat and warm chest for chest congestion, peace and love for anger, and coolness in hot areas. 3) Imagine the body free of pain and healthy. 4) Pat yourself on the back and tell yourself that you have done a good job of eliminating the condition. This technique has been used for anxiety, asthma, headache, viruses, to enhance the quality of life, and to reduce pain and stress.

Another exercise that can be used to reduce stress in any situation is: Close your eyes and as you inhale imagine yourself as a balloon filling with air. On each breath you become fuller and fuller. When you become completely full imagine the air leaving the balloon and the tension you feel going with it.

Research on Visualization

Richardson et al (1997) found imagery useful in the treatment of cancer patients. Gruber (1993) found similar results. Simonton (1980) found that when 225 breast cancer patients received a variety of interventions including imagery their median survival time was extended. Scott et al (1986) found that visualization would help alleviate nausea and vomiting associated with chemotherapy for cancer. Several researchers (Borysenko, 1987; Siegel, 1986; and Simonton et al, 1978) found that visualization helped mobilize the immune system in patients with cancer. Rider (1990) found that imagery could improve the immune system functioning of normal college students when compared with students who did not receive this intervention. Albright (1990) found imagery useful in reducing pain. Using patients who previously were trained in biofeedback, he found that using warming imagery decreased sensitivity to pressure and also increased muscle relaxation and skin temperature. Walco et al (1992) also found imagery was effective in reducing pain in children with arthritis when used in combination with progressive relaxation, and meditative breathing. Holden-Lund (1988) found visualization decreased post-op anxiety; Daake and Gueldner (1989) and Manyande et al (1991) found it decreased post-op pain; and Fazio (1996) and Rapkin et al (1991) found it decreased hospital stays after surgery. Ievleva and Orlick (1991) found that visualization speeded the healing process of injuries in subjects with knee and ankle injuries. Moody et al (1993) found that guided imagery significantly improved the perceived quality of life in older subjects with moderate bronchitis and emphysema. Alternative Medicine (1994) concluded that some studies on imagery have been well controlled and other have reported single cases or small groups, However, the overriding conclusions are that there is a relationship between imagery of body changes and actual body changes. Closely related to visualization are exercises that help us replace negative attitudes and thoughts with positive ones having a positive effect on health.

Working with Your Attitudes and Thoughts

Exercises that work with your attitudes and thoughts and may be effective in reducing stress and improving health are discussed now.

Thought Stopping.

This technique stops repetitive stressful thoughts. Practice this for 3 to 7 days until the repetitive thought has stopped. Process: 1) Close your eyes. 2) Choose a stressful thought such as the fear of flying. 3) Bring the thought to your attention. 4) Imagine a situation where the thought is likely to occur – such as when flying. 5) Interrupt the thought with an alarm, a snapping of your fingers, or repeating the word "stop". 6) Replace the negative thought with a positive one. For example, imagine looking out the window and thinking, "It's a beautiful view from here," instead of fearing the situation.

Change Attitudes and Thoughts.

Replace negative with positive thoughts or remain positive. In this exercise you replace each negative thought with a positive one throughout the day. If you are driving and someone cuts in front of you bless him or her and wish him or her a great day instead of the usual response. You will find that as you practice this daily for a period of time you become much more positive in your reactions to situations and people and life become less stressful. You may also want to fill you mind with positive thoughts so there is no room for negative ones. This can be done well in combination with affirmations.

Continual Positive Thoughts

Fill your mind with so many positive thoughts there is no room for negative ones. When you wake in the morning think, "What a wonderful day – I feel so great today – I look forward to being at work with my colleagues," and other positive thoughts. Reinforce positive thoughts throughout the day. If you have a negative thought, immediately replace it with a positive one. For example, if a coworker friend who you usually eat lunch with ignores you and goes to lunch with someone else wish him or her a great lunch and proceed to lunch alone or with another coworker. Think to yourself, it is good to converse with someone else and get new ideas. As you continue to fill your mind with positive thoughts, there will be no room for negative thoughts. Then you will attract positive people and positive health. (What you send out returns to you or like attracts like.) Affirmations may be useful in this process of staying positive and replacing negative thoughts with positive ones. Eventually you will find that your thoughts are almost always positive and you will be amazed at the effect this has on your life. I CHALLENGE YOU TO TRY THIS. It is also important when you are working with these exercises and attitude changes to avoid negative people, if possible. They tend to reinforce negative thoughts.

Closely related to these mental processes of remaining positive and changing negative thoughts is the spiritual outlook of optimism. Because it is so closely related it will be discussed here instead of under spiritual concepts.

Optimism – Remaining Positive

Optimism has been shown to be effective in increasing health and preventing illness. When my mother was diagnosed with cancer of the cervix of the uterus in 1949 she went to the hospital knowing the family did not expect her to live. When she returned home in remission her family doctor told her he had not expected her to live to get to the hospital that was about 200 miles away. She replied, "I had to come home because I have three children in school yet, and I need to see that they graduate from high school." She was optimistic of her recovery and of living to see her children through school. She remained optimistic and lived for about 40 more years.

Optimism and a positive outlook was part of my self-treatment when I was diagnosed with lung cancer in 1974. My doctor told me I would be dead within 6 months without surgery that I refused and instead used a variety of alternative treatments. An important aspect of my treatment was to remain positive and optimistic. One organization that assists individuals to develop an optimistic outlook on life is the Optimist Club. Their creed reflects their philosophy. This philosophy tells us a lot about how to develop optimism. Basically it involves having faith in ourselves, in God, and in others. All of the exercises under spiritual and many of those under mental such as affirmations, remaining positive and changing negative thoughts to positive ones will help develop optimism.

Research on Positive Thoughts and Optimism

Justice (1988) found that people who are optimistic and confident come through medical procedures in better condition and have less mortality and morbidity than those who are less hopeful and less confident. Kamen-Siegel et al (1991) found that optimism influences the immune system in a positive way. In his study of elderly people, those who were pessimistic and lacked hope had a lower ratio of T-helper cells to T-suppressor cells and had poorer T-lymphocyte response when the immune system was challenged. Martin Seligman confirmed these results in his study of 300 elderly patients with an average age of 71. Likewise, Ranard (1989) obtained the same findings in a group of healthy elderly subjects. He concluded that hopeful people have a more robust immune system.

Friedman et al (1992) found that enthusiastic people tend to be the most resilient, self-healing people and enthusiasm is correlated with recovery from illness. On the other hand, Shekelle et al (1983) found that chronic hostility has a negative effect on health. In his study of 1875 working men between age 40 and 55, high levels of hostility correlated with higher death rates including death from cardiovascular disease.

Affirmations

Affirmations can be used to help you remain positive, to replace negative thoughts with positive ones, or to improve you're self-esteem. All reduce stress. Both Louise Hay (1984) in *You Can Heal Your Life* and Anne Marie Evers in *Affirmations: Your Passport to Happiness and Much More* discuss affirmations in detail. Louise Hay offers examples of affirmations for various conditions and situations and Anne Marie presents a process that one uses with affirmations to obtain what they want in life. She says all affirmations are successful if they are done correctly.

Affirmations are discussed briefly here. One affirmation that is useful to build self-esteem and presented by Louise Hay involves saying non-stop, "I approve of myself... I approve of myself." She also says you can look into the mirror and say, "[your name], I love you just as you are." Repeat this regularly. For increased wealth use affirmations such as, "Riches of all sorts are drawn to me," or "I am a magnet for divine prosperity." For more friends use, "Love is everywhere and I am loving and loveable." To improve a relationship with the boss, "I have a wonderful boss who is always trying to make things easier for me."

Affirmations should be present oriented with "I am" or "I have" statements instead of future oriented ones starting with "I will have" or "I want". Future oriented affirmations are never attainable because our subconscious mind will keep them out of reach. Some affirmations that may be useful for you to start a change process in your lives are: "I am the right size and weight for me"; "I am happy and healthy at my ideal weight"; "I am attractive at the ideal weight I have obtained" (for weight loss); "I am a wonderful person who has many friends"; "I am a loving person surrounded by love" (for lonely people); "I have a wonderful, fulfilling job", "I have a wonderful boss and coworkers who support and respect me" (for those who want to improve relations at work) , and "I am finishing this race easily." With these guidelines in mind, you should be able to develop your own affirmations. If you need help consult one of the books identified above.

Energy Exercises

Donna Eden and others have developed a system of treating the body that uses your body's energy to boost your stamina and vitality. Some exercises are specific for stress. These will be briefly reviewed here based upon her work. The interested reader is referred to *Energy Medicine* authored by Donna Eden and published by Penguin Putnam, Inc in New York City (pp 87–91).

It is possible to reprogram your autonomic nervous system so you do not respond to daily stresses. To develop this ability start by remembering stressful situations from the past and then hold two neurovascular points on your forehead. This process conditions the brain to have a composed reaction instead of a crises response. The points are above the eyes on the forehead where there is a bump or raised area. Place your fingertips on these areas with your thumbs on your temples next to your eyes and breathe deeply. Continue for a few minutes (3 to 5). Repeat this daily until the memory of the incident no longer evokes a crises response. Then use it when new stressors impinge upon you until you are reprogrammed to not react in a stressful way.

There are other exercises that will release pent up stress. Three of these follow and additional ones can be found on page 91 in Eden's book. **Expel the Venom** is useful when you feel angry or judgmental and takes a minute or two to complete. Begin with your hands on your hips with fingers spread. Take a deep breath. As you exhale make a Shhhhhhhhhh sound like telling someone to be quiet. As you inhale deeply swing your arms out and then circle high above your head. Turn your palms so they are facing you and make a fist. Exhale loudly and make the Shhhhhhhh sound dropping your fisted hand and opening them as you near your thigh. Repeat until the anger leaves.

In the **crown pull** you refresh the mind and release mental congestion. Begin by placing your thumbs on your temples on the side of your head and your fingertips just above the center of your eyebrows. The four fingers may extend from your eyebrows to your hairline. Slowly and using slight pressure pull your fingers toward your temples so you stretch the skin above the eyebrows. Repeat at the center of the forehead; at the hairline; at the top of your head; and over the curve of the back of your head. Repeat each stretch one or two times.

The **Wayne Cook Exercise** helps you focus your mind better and think more clearly. Start with your right foot over your left knee and wrap your left hand around your right ankle and your hand around the ball of your right foot. Breathe in slowly and pull your leg toward you to create a stretch. Breathe out of your mouth and let your body relax. Repeat 4 or 5 times. Repeat with the opposite foot in the same position and with the breathing exercises for 4 or 5 times. Then uncross your legs and form a pyramid with your fingertips and hands. Put your thumbs on your 3rd eye and inhale slowly through your nose and exhale through your mouth. Inhale again through your nose and separate your thumbs slowly across your forehead pulling the skin. Bring the thumbs back to the third eye and then bring your hand in front of you putting them together in a prayer position while breathing deeply. This should take about 2 minutes.

Meditation
Introduction

Meditation is a positive process used by the author during his cancer regime as part of a holistic approach for recovery from lung cancer and since recovery to prevent a recurrence. Although it is placed under the mental category it could also be considered a spiritual intervention. Cayce (Study Group of the Association for Research and Enlightenment, 1942) says meditation is "the emptying of ourselves of all that hinders the Creative Force from rising along the natural channels of our physical bodies to be disseminated through the sensitive spiritual centers in our physical bodies." Meditation means putting away the worries and concerns of the day and emptying the mind so that God can speak to us. Cayce makes the distinction between meditation and prayer by saying that in prayer we speak to God, and in meditation God speaks to us. Meditation can be thought of as a process of achieving awareness without thought.

The Process

The meditation process involves preparation and implementation. Preparation may vary from person to person. You may try out and decide on one or more of the following activities to purify the physical and mental bodies before coming in contact with the creative force in meditation. Some individuals choose to cleanse the physical body with soap and water; some avoid certain foods before meditation; and some choose to perform relaxation exercises or deep breathing. Some useful breathing and head and neck exercises were presented earlier.

Some people like sounds as part of the preparation so they

play music such as Gregorian chants before meditating whereas others prefer to chant themselves. Still others like to experience the sensation of smell and will burn incense before and during meditation. My own personal preference is to play Gregorian chants and burn sandalwood incense, whereas chanting alone or in a group makes me uncomfortable.

Next it is important to decide if you want to meditate with others or alone. Some like to meditate with others especially when they are beginning. Two useful groups that may be available to the reader are the Friends Quaker Church and an Edgar Cayce Study Group. The traditional Quaker church holds silent services on Sundays during which members meditate until the spirit moves them and then they stand and speak. There is no minister at these services. So if you find a traditional Quaker church in your area you may want to attend a service and make up your mind about returning. The author personally found this a wonderful group of people and a great group to meditate with.

The Edgar Cayce Study Groups (Search for God groups) meet in numerous locations throughout the United States and world. At weekly meetings members meditate together and study materials developed with Edgar Cayce when he was alive that focus on reading about and using the spiritual attributes of patience, love, forgiveness and others to become better people. Usually a group will select a discipline to practice each week related to the material being read and discussed and will report back on the successes and failures of the practice selected. They also select a time when members will meditate daily with their group members while each is in his/her own home. This experience is invaluable to those interested in a better spiritual life and better health. If interested in trying this approach, contact the study group office at the Association for Research and Enlightenment in Virginia Beach to locate a study group near you.

There are different types of meditation and consequently

different processes but the following is the one the author has used over the past 43 years. It is the Edgar Cayce approach and the author believes his experience in Search for God groups and meditation seems to combine the best aspects of all types of meditation from a spiritual point of view. One of the first hurdles for the person new to meditation is to sit quietly for a period of time without thinking of the day's activities. We are conditioned to being active and it is difficult to sit. Then when we do sit we are conditioned to thinking about everything from what happened today to planning for tomorrow. Or our emotions take over and we worry about an encounter from the day or unfinished tasks for tomorrow. Thus, it is helpful to meditate at the same time and in the same place daily to facilitate the process of sitting quietly and quieting the mind.

Some people like to sit and others prefer to lie down while meditating. Some sit in the lotus position whereas others sit in a chair in a relaxed position with the spine erect. Some sit with their palms facing upwards whereas others hold their hands in a relaxed position. Do whatever is comfortable for you. I prefer to sit in a relaxed position with the spine erect and hands resting comfortably on my lap.

Next, focus on an affirmation, passage from the Bible or some other inspirational words to focus your mind. In the Search for God books used by study groups, there is an affirmation for each chapter that relates to the material being discussed. These are closely related to biblical passages. Some found in these books are "Lo, I am with you always, Even till the End", or "Be Still, And Know that I am God", or "Not my Will but Thine Oh Lord". Those who practice Transcendental Meditation are given a mantra to use.

Next, empty your mind of all thoughts so that "God may speak with you". When you begin thinking again or experience emotions refocus your mind on the affirmation until you have stilled the mind and can return to the state of an empty mind.

Continue for at least 20 minutes. Some people meditate 20 minutes twice a day. Some meditate daily for 30 minutes. After you have mastered the sitting and emptying of the mind, you will choose a time period that is comfortable for you. With practice you will be able to sit, quickly empty your mind and enjoy the refreshing feeling that occurs following the meditation. The author meditates for at least 30 minutes regularly each evening before bedtime and occasionally in the morning.

Research on Meditation

Over 600 scientific studies have been carried out on Transcendental Meditation. Review these on the Internet site (www.tm.org) under the research tab. A brief overview of these findings follows: Over a two-year period one study reported a significant increase in intelligence of one group of university students who meditated over another who did not. Another study showed a significant increase in creativity on the Torrance Test of Creative Thinking among students who meditated over a matched control group who did not. Over 375 studies were reviewed in one published analysis and they consistently showed that those who meditated were significantly more effective in producing improvements in self-esteem and decreasing anxiety than any other technique used for self-improvement.

These studies also showed an improvement in physical health. In one study of blood pressure results of groups over 3 months, the systolic and diastolic pressure dropped by 10.6 and 5.9 mm Hg in the group of meditators, and 4.0 and 2.1 mm Hg in the PMR (progressive muscle relaxation) group, and there was no change in the usual care group. In another study using random assignments to control or study groups where the initial serum level of blood cholesterol were the same, the Transcendental Meditation group dropped to 225 with a plus or minus 9.4 mg/100ml compared to their own baseline. The controls remained at the baseline of 259 with a plus or minus of 8.9 mg/100 ml. Another study looked at medical utilization and found that it decreased by 50% for meditators compared to a matched control group. A 2006 study (Schneider et al) concluded, "the use of the TM technique may be effective in improving the quality of life and functional capacity of heart failure patients." In another study (Rainforth et al, 2007) published a meta-analysis of 17 published studies from the medical literature that were selected from over 100 published studies for their careful experimental design utilizing randomised controlled trials. They reported on the effects of stress reduction techniques on elevated blood pressure in about 1000 subjects. The treatments employed were simple biofeedback, relaxation-assisted biofeedback, progressive muscle relaxation, stress management training, and the Transcendental Meditation program. Results showed none of the treatment approaches demonstrated statistically significant reductions in elevated blood pressure except the Transcendental Meditation program that showed both significant clinical and statistical reductions in blood pressure.

McSherry (1990) and Orme-Johnson (1987) compared a group of 2000 meditators with 600,000 non-meditators and found that insurance statistics showed meditators used 30 to 87% less medical care than non-meditators in all but one (childbirth) of the 18 categories. Alternative Medicine (1994) reported that clients at the Harvard Community Health Plan who attended a six-week group including meditation had significantly fewer physician visits during the following six months at an average saving of $171 per client. In another study long-term meditators were found to be physiologically 12 years younger than their chronological age.

The website identified earlier summarizes findings from over 500 research studies conducted over the past 25 years at more than 200 independent universities and research centers in over 30 countries. These studies show that meditation has a total effect on a person's mind, body, environment and behavior. Specifically these results show that meditation: 1) increases happiness; 2) reduces stress; 3) reduces elevated blood pressure; 4) improves relationships; 5) increases energy; 6) reduces insomnia; 7) increases intelligence; 8) improves memory; 9) improves health; 10) reverses biological aging; and 11) improves the quality of life in society. The interested reader should complete a Google search for additional information and references.

Spiritual

Some concepts mentioned throughout the book include praying for others who are difficult, developing spiritual attributes, serving others, and working with ideals. Exercises related to these and other spiritual concepts will be presented now.

Pray For Others Who are Difficult

Closely related to changing attitudes from negative to positive discussed earlier are the techniques of praying for others with whom you have a problem. In this exercise: 1) Identify someone with whom you have a disagreement or whom you dislike. 2) Pray for that person daily for one week. Pray for health and prosperity and the best in life for him/her. 3) After one week evaluate how you feel about the person. Often, it will seem like he/she has become more likeable., However, it is likely that you have changed in your feelings.

And as you change your attitude you will move to a higher level of thinking and feeling that will be reflected in your inter-actions and that person will respond to the new (in progress) you. This is effective in improving relationships but also has a health effect because in combination with other interventions discussed here you are less likely to feel and express anger, resentment or some other negative emotions that are known to affect health and increase your stress reaction.

Research on Prayer

There have been multiple studies on the effects of prayer on healing and health. Some of these include the following. In a study in 2000, Astin et al analyzed 23 clinical studies (over 2,700 patients) that examined the effects of prayer, spiritual healing and other unconventional treatment on patients' health. They defined spiritual healing as "a broad classification of approaches involving the intentional influence of one or more persons upon another living system without using physical means of intervention;" and Distant Healing as "a conscious act that attempts to benefit another person's physical or emotional well-being at a distance." They found over 100 studies on prayer and healing but selected only 23 that utilized appropriate research techniques to increase the validity such as randomization, double-blind techniques, were clinical, were on humans, and were published in peer-reviewed journals. Over half of these studies (13 studies and 57%) found a positive impact on patients from these interventions. Nine studies showed no effect, and one showed a negative effect. The highest percentage of positive results was found in studies in which spiritual healing was used, especially where the healer treated the energy field around the patient's body. In this intervention the healer most often used his hands on the energy field in a technique called therapeutic touch. For this intervention 7 of the 11 studies were positive. Other interventions included distant healing by prayer. The authors concluded that the results warranted further study of distant healing. Mercola (1999) reported on a study in which 1000 heart patients were prayed for without their knowledge. All patients received standard health care but half of the patients were prayed for by 15 teams of 5 self-identified individuals who pray. The prayed-for group had an 11% reduction in medical complications or the need for surgery while in the hospital compared to those who did not receive prayer. Braud (1994) reviewed several additional studies on the effect of distant and close prayer on healing and found comparable results.

A classic study by Comstock and Partridge (1972) of 91,909 people living in Maryland found churchgoers who attended services at least once weekly had significantly lower death rates for the following conditions: 50% reduction in coronary artery disease; 56% reduction in emphysema; 74% reduction in cirrhosis of the liver; and a 53% reduction in suicide. Koenig et al (1994) found that people with a strong religious commitment are less likely to turn to alcoholism.

Matthews and Clark (1998) say that in 75% of 325 studies of different types the findings indicated that involvement in religious activities benefited health and well-being. Although they did not establish a cause-effect relationship, they strongly supported an important connection between religious practices and good health. Matthews, Lawson, and Barry (1993) in their four-volume bibliography summarize the benefits of religious involvement. A Google search will provide many studies on the relationship of prayer and healing, stress, and good health.

Developing Spiritual Attributes

Incorporating spiritual attributes into one's life reduces stress and has a powerful effect on health and relationships. Exercises to develop some important ones follow such as faith, forgiveness, and serving others.

Faith

"Faith is being sure of what we hope for and certain of what we do not see" Hebrews 11:1. What is faith? It is "an attribute of the soul. It is the inner spiritual knowledge of the Creative Force of the universe" (Study Group of the Association for Research and Enlightenment, 1942). It is the "confident assurance that something we want is going to happen. It is the certainty that what we hope for is waiting for us, even though we cannot see it up ahead (The Living Bible, Paraphrased, 1973). The story of

Noah in the Bible is an example of faith. When Noah heard God's warning, he believed it even though there were no signs of flooding. Because of his faith and actions, he was prepared when flooding occurred. When I do not get what I think I want at the moment I know that God has something better in mind for me and eventually it will unfold. That is also faith.

Faith relates to God, to ourselves and to our fellow beings. The opposite of faith is doubt and when we doubt ourselves we doubt the God within. When we doubt our fellow being, we are not looking for the best in him/her which should be our ideal. Doubt is closely related to the negative feelings of fear and worry. Worry is a result of fear. And fear, in turn, is a result of doubt. The opposite of doubt is faith. In Luke 12:22-25 the Bible says: "What is the use of worrying? What good does it do? Will it add a single day to your life? Of course it will not. And if worry can't even do such little things as that, what's the use of worrying about the bigger things."

Faith cannot be taught or developed from reading about it. Faith is developed by using it and experiencing positive results. The exercises below may help the interested reader begin or further develop this important spiritual attribute.

Faith Exercises

Before we can replace worry and doubt with faith it is necessary to be aware of situations in our lives in which it occurs. Once identified we can change our worry habits by replacing these negative thoughts with positive ones such as "God is with me and looking out for me and bringing whatever is best for me." You will recognize this as a positive affirmation. Through an ongoing process of analyzing worry situations and replacing the negative thoughts with positive ones you can build faith. The following exercises follow this format:

Exercise I: 1) Make a list of all experiences in which you used faith. 2) Analyze the factors that influenced your faith at these times. 3) How did you feel after the experience was over? 4) Have you repeated the use of faith in similar situations?

Exercise II: 1) Look at your past and find experiences where you did not have faith. 2) Relive one experience. 3) Replace the lack of faith with faith in the situation. 4) How would you react in the same situation in the future?

Exercise III: 1) Think of a situation in which you felt anxious and worried such as: a) fear of job loss; b) fear of loss of a significant relationship; c) money worries; or d) other concerns. 2) Relive the situations including the feelings you experienced. 3) Now replace the feeling with faith or knowing that God will bring only the best to you. 4) Would you have faith in a similar situation in the future?

Exercise IV: 1) In the next week be consciously aware of situations in which doubt and worry creep into your thoughts. 2) Immediately replace that thought with a knowing that God is looking out for you and will bring only the best to you. What ever happens is for your greatest good and ultimate happiness. 3) Were you successful in replacing negative with positive thoughts? 4) How did you feel? 5) You are beginning to experience faith. Pat yourself on the back for a successful effort.

Worry may also be a result of self-centeredness that may lead to isolation from others. Thus, concern for and assisting others will take your mind off your own worries. The following activities to overcome self-centeredness may help you replace doubt with faith when used in combination with the other exercises above.

Think about what interests you. 1) Are you interested in politics? Helping sick people? Helping the elderly? Developing spiritually? Getting in better physical shape? 2) Select one area of interest and get involved – join a political action group; volunteer for meals on wheels, in a nursing home, or a hospital; join a church, spiritual study group or optimistic group such as the ARE study group or the optimist club; or join the YMCA health club, or Weight Watchers.

Forgiveness

Forgiving others not only improves relationships, it also improves health and reduces stress. The following exercise may help you develop forgiveness.

Exercise:

1) Think back about a particular situation that was hurtful to you.
2) See the particular situation from the other person's point of view.
3) Recognize that there are times when we hurt others also.
4) Acknowledge that the past cannot be changed and accept responsibility for your own healing of the situation.
5) Don't expect an apology because forgiveness does not equal reconciliation.
6) Wish the other person well and send good thoughts.
7) Congratulate yourself for the positive action you have taken. You will feel like a weight has been lifted from your shoulders.

Research

In one study carried out in 2000, 71 people relived hurtful memories and added two different endings: 1) harboring the grudge; or 2) forgiving the person involved. Common offenses among friends, parents, siblings and romantic partners included betrayal of trust, rejection, lying, and insults. Measurement of heart rates, blood pressure, perspiration, and subjective emotions showed that heart rates and blood pressure were 2½ times lower when participants forgave than when they held grudges. In addition, those holding onto the grudge sweat more and felt more negative, sad, and angry.

Service to Others

Jesus advocated being of service to others. This spiritual practice improves your health and reduces stress when positive spiritual ideals and motives underlie this service.

Here service to others is separated into community services that emphasize service to groups, and service to individuals that emphasize daily service to individuals.

How can you serve others in the community? A) Select one or more of the following opportunities: 1) volunteer in a hospital; 2) a nursing home; 3) for meals on wheels; 4) in a homeless shelter; 5) an officer in your homeowners' association; 6) be active in a political party; 7) an advocacy group; 8) be active in a professional or service organizations; 9) other organizations. B) Devote some time every week or two to one or more of these activities. C) Serve other people, as you believe Jesus would serve them. D) Evaluate your successes and failures after each time in the community. E) Use visualization to relive the failures and replace them with a positive outcome. F) Pat yourself on the back for your efforts and successes.

How can you serve others as individuals? I think of a friend who is a waitress and who says she likes her job because it allows her to talk with and be of service to others. She is always talking with her customers, offering comfort, patting them on the back for a job well done and other behaviors that shows that she truly cares about herself, others, and God.

Are you cheerful and helpful to others or is it a job and a task to get through the day? Do you feel tired after the day is over? Are you worried, afraid or have other negative feelings? If so, something is wrong with your approach to life and needs to be changed. Try the following for one week. 1) Be consciously aware of your interactions with others during your working and leisure hours. 2) Did you offer a smile to all whom you contacted? Did you greet everyone in a friendly way? Did you maintain eye contact? Did you offer comforting reassurance when indicated?

Were your conversations positive and upbeat? Did you touch in a comforting, reassuring way, when indicated? Did you feel good about your interactions? 3) Evaluate each day and identify your successes and failures. 4) Use visualization and prayer or other exercises such as positive affirmations, if appropriate, to imagine a different outcome for your failures. For example, if you have problems with superiors and coworkers, positive affirmations and prayer can be very effective to bring about change. 5) Try out your new visualized behaviors in subsequent interactions. 6) Pat yourself on the back for your successes. 7) Evaluate how you feel when leaving work after a week.

Ideals

Before individuals can change and permanently improve their lives they may also need to work with their ideals that, in turn, influence health, relationships, and stress levels. An ideal is something we live with daily and is our motivating force. It is our life direction that motivates our attitudes and behavior. Thus, spiritual ideals are manifest in the mental (attitude) and result in the physical (behavior).

Ideals may be conscious or unconscious and spiritual or non-spiritual. Ideals reside in a higher realm than thought and may or may not be attuned to the spirit of the creator-God, Allah, or some other identified higher force. For example, selfish thoughts result from selfish motives and may be manifest in jealousy, anger or other emotions that lead to negative behavior. On the other hand, spiritual ideals that are attuned to the creator lead to patience, forgiveness, love, kindness, and compassion and are manifest in positive behaviors toward others. Positive spiritual attributes are effective in reducing stress whereas negative ones may increase it.

Ideas and Ideals

Individuals often confuse ideas with ideals. Ideas tend to be human thoughts (things) that you own whereas ideals are attributes that own and influence you. For example, those who try to force their religion onto others with a "You must believe" attitude have confused ideals with human ideas. These are their thoughts that they own or possess. We have many ideas about God, Jesus, Allah and others we have learned and use in our life. These ideas are like possessions that belong to us and that we use with others. However, ideals are not possessions that we own. Instead, ideals own us in order to become effective in our lives. For example, until we allow love, forgiveness and patience to take over our lives and influence our thoughts and actions we have not accepted these spiritual ideals.

Identifying and Specifying Your Ideals

Initially we should try to discover our ideals. Take some time at the end of each day to reflect on experiences that you remember. Write down what you thought about or did in each experience. Then write down the conscious or unconscious force that may have motivated the thoughts or behavior. For example, did you get mad at someone and speak in an angry or rude way. The force that directed the behavior might have been resentment you had been holding toward that person. On the other hand, you might have been helpful to another person and the force motivating this behavior might have been an especially good meditation in which you asked to be of service to others. As you write down your experiences and the possible forces behind them, you are specifying what your ideals may have been. You may also be aware that ideals vary from experience to experience.

Ideals can be identified as spiritual, mental and physical. Because spiritual ideals are manifest in the mental and physical activities, and the body, mind, and spirit are recognized as a whole, it is useful to begin by identifying and writing spiritual ideals for your life in order to improve your health and relationships and thereby reduce stress. During prayer and/or meditation each day, it is helpful to reflect on the qualities that you are most aware of that you would like to have directing your life. During your quiet time at the end of the week, reflect on these qualities and integrate them into one spiritual ideal such as 'love', 'peace', 'God', or 'oneness'.

Applying Identified Ideals

Exercises may also assist in improving mental and physical ideals. Reaffirm the spiritual ideal you have identified above. Then pick an area of your life you want to improve and identify mental ideals (thoughts and feelings), and physical ideals (activities) that apply. Areas for improvement might be diet, exercise regime, personal relationships, or professional relationships at the workplace. Mental ideals identified may suggest physical ideals. For example, in an effort to improve a relationship a mental attitude of caring might suggest inviting a friend to dinner or telephoning regularly.

Sometimes others try to influence our thoughts and these efforts may be consistent with or against our ideals. For example, others may encourage idle gossiping that is against our spiritual ideal of love for all. We should be true to our ideals even when it means standing alone. Each day we should evaluate the day and be aware of the ways others have tried to influence our decisions. Next, determine whether or not we went along with them in order to avoid disagreement even if it was against our ideals. Then replay the experience in your mind and identify how you could be kind and sensitive to the opinions and ideas of others but also make your decisions based upon your ideals. These exercises will improve your relationships and have a positive effect on health.

Parts of this chapter were reproduced and modified from Helvie, C. (2007) *Healthy Holistic Aging*, Minneapolis, Minnesota: Syren Books with permission.

About the Author

Carl O. Helvie, RN, DrPH is a nationally recognized health practitioner and widely published author who has developed multiple strategies for healthy holistic aging and holistic health in his clinical work as a nursing practitioner, educator, and radio host for the Holistic Health Show.

Applying these concepts in his life he is now age 79 and free of chronic illnesses and prescribed medications being one of the few who escaped the statistics of 3 chronic illnesses and 5 prescribed medications for a 75 year old.

Dr. Helvie began his career in 1951 when he entered nursing school at St. Lawrence State Hospital, School of Nursing in upstate New York, completed the program and passed his boards as a registered nurse. Thereafter, he completed a baccalaureate in nursing (New York University), followed by master's degrees in public health nursing (University of California) and public health/mental health (Johns Hopkins University, School of Public Health); and a doctorate in public health/mental health (Johns Hopkins University).

His career spans 58 years and included functioning as a nurse practitioner, educator, researcher, and author. Besides staff and head nursing at Bellevue Hospital in New York City, he functioned as a staff nurse at the Monroe County Hospital in Rochester, New York, and the VA Hospital in San Francisco, California. Thereafter, he was a public health nurse in Oakland and San Francisco, California before entering academia. He taught graduate and undergraduate nursing students and health students at Old Dominion University, and previously mental health nursing graduate students at Duke University, and undergraduate public health nursing students at the University of California in San Francisco. During his years in education he authored 9 books and book chapters, 56 articles in professional journals , and 55 research papers presented around the United States and Europe. One of the highlights of his career was receiving a grant from the Division of Nursing for almost $1 million dollars and establishing and administering a compre- hensive health care program for chronic and acute illnesses among homeless and low-income people in an eastern city in the United States. This experience culminated in a book written with colleagues from Europe and Russia on *Homelessness in the United States, Europe, and Russia*. Another highlight of his career was developing an *Energy Theory of Nursing and Health* that was utilized with graduate and undergraduate nursing students and refining and incorporating it into his books over a 25-year period. The theory in now used in several graduate programs, included in nursing books, and used as a framework for a research book in the United States and used in a research project in Taiwan. Dr. Helvie was recognized in many national references including Outstanding Educator in America, Who's Who, Who's Who in Virginia, and Who's Who in American Nursing. He also was awarded the Distinguished Career in Public Health Award by the American Public Health Association in 1999.

One of his memorable life experiences was being diagnosed with lung cancer in 1974 and being given 6 months to live. Choosing to forgo traditional therapy and using alternative inter- ventions instead he is alive and healthy 38 years later. This experience not only brought him closer to God but also provided an opportunity to encourage and assist others in a similar situation.

Since retiring from academia at age 69 as Professor Emeritus of Nursing, Dr. Helvie has continued to remain active. In 2003 he taught a summer course on community health nursing at the University of Applied Sciences in Frankfurt, Germany and then traveled as a consultant to Moscow, Russia. In 2007 he published his 7th book that was on *Healthy Holistic Aging* and was inter- viewed on 45 radio shows on this topic. He also began his free online monthly newsletter on Healthy Holistic Aging and in 2008 he began hosting the Holistic Health Show on BBS Radio. He now has a large following on his radio show and receives many emails monthly from others who have been diagnosed with cancer and who ask for assistance locating resources for alternative treatment. These email are always a priority and encouragement and resources are provided. Dr. Helvie finds his life intellectually stimulating and personally rewarding and plans to continue helping others as long as he is healthy and able to do so. More information is available at: www.HolisticHealthShow.com

About the Contributors

Dr. Francisco Contreras serves as director, president and chairman of the Oasis of Hope Hospital. A distinguished oncologist and surgeon, Contreras is renowned for combining conventional and alternative medical treatments with emotional and spiritual support to provide patients with the most positive treatment experience possible. He passionately integrates the healing power of faith, hope and love with his patients and educates them with the Biblical principles of health.

Oasis of Hope was founded by Contreras' father, Dr. Ernesto Contreras, Sr. in 1963, and since then the hospital has provided integrative cancer treatment for more than 100,000 patients. As director, Contreras continues the practice of his father's two fundamental principles – do no harm and treat the patient as yourself. Today, Contreras oversees the treatment of 800 cancer patients annually.

After graduating with honors from medical school at the Autonomous University of Mexico in Toluca, Contreras studied alternative therapy at the Oasis of Hope Hospital. He then completed his specialty in surgical oncology at the University of Vienna in Austria, where he also graduated with honors.

Contreras has authored and co-authored several books concerning integrative therapy, cancer and heart disease prevention and chronic illness, including *Beating Cancer, The Hope of Living Cancer Free, A Healthy Heart, The Hope of Living Long and Well*, and *Dismantling Cancer*.

In addition to writing for numerous medical journals, Contreras has participated in medical conferences such as the World Conference on Breast Cancer and is active in the Cancer Control Society. He has been interviewed on CNN, MSNBC, Fox News, and most major Christian networks. He has been a part of governmental organizations, including the Georgia House of

Representatives Health Policy Task Force and the Japanese Medical Association. He has also been on special assignment to Slovakia as a member of the Mexican Health Advisory Board.

A qualified entry-level professional motorcycle racer, Contreras says that racing is similar to performing surgery in that it requires 100% focus. Contreras and his wife, Rosa, have four daughters, one son and one granddaughter. The family attends church in Bonita, California, and enjoys skiing and travel. **More information is available at: www.Oasisof Hope.com**

Kim Dalzell, PhD, RD, LD, has helped people fight cancer with nutrition for over twenty years. She has appeared on countless television and radio programs and is an advisory board member for Lifetime Television's Health Corner show and Breast Cancer Wellness magazine. She has served as spokesperson for Cancer Treatment Centers of America and wrote the foreword for *The Recipe for Breast Cancer* – a first-of-its-kind nutrition and cancer book in Japan. Her award-winning book *Challenge Cancer and Win!* has been translated into Japanese and adapted into a distance learning course. Her presentations create laughter and learning. You can learn more about Dr. Kim's speaking and consultation services at www.naturesanswerto-cancer.com.

Dr. James Wm. Forsythe is described as a 'Renaissance' man and practices Integrative Medical Oncology and Anti-Aging medicine. He is the only Board Certified Medical Oncologist with certification in Homeopathic Medicine in the United States. Dr. Forsythe received his Doctorate of Medicine from University of California, San Francisco in 1964. He received his under-graduate degree from University of California at Berkeley. He is Board Certified in Internal Medicine, Medical Oncology and Utilization Review and Quality Assurance. He is certified in Homeopathy. He is a former Associate Professor at the University of Nevada Medical School. He is a retired Full

Colonel, former State Surgeon in the Nevada Army National Guard, and served in Vietnam where he received a commendation medal. He is the owner and medical director of Century Wellness Clinic, which incorporates integrative medical treatments for all adult cancers. He has been involved with clinical outcome based cancer studies with integrative treatment therapies. These include clinical studies on paw paw, Poly-MVA, and an ongoing study that includes all his integrative treatment modulates. The studies have all shown improved efficacy over conventional therapies. In 2001 he started to incorporate preventative medicine after years of treating cancer patients to help the aging population manage chronic disease. He prescribed Human Growth Hormone therapy for adult deficiencies. He also included BHRT into his protocol. In 2005 the FDA raided his home and clinic at gun point because he was using Human Growth Hormone 'off-label'. In 2006 he was indicted by a Federal District Court of Nevada. In 2007 under the counsel of Mirch & Mirch he went to trial and became the only physician in the history of the United States to be tried in front of a Federal District Court jury for off-label use of a drug, HGH. He was found Not Guilty. Dr. Forsythe has developed a National Protocol under the sponsorship of the FDA for Age Related Adult Growth Hormone Deficiency Syndrome. Dr. Forsythe is a world-renowned lecturer and author. He authored and co-authored numerous books and his most recent books include: *Anti-Aging Cures* and *Take Control of Your Cancer*. He co-authored, *The Ultimate Guide to Natural Health*. Dr. Forsythe also has been a contributing author to Suzanne Somers' top sellers: *Knockout: Interviews with Doctors Who Are Curing Cancer – And How to Prevent Getting It in the First Place* **and** *Breakthrough: Eight Steps to Wellness*. Dr. Forsythe has been a co-author in Burton Goldberg's books on alternative medicine. Dr. Forsythe is owner and Medical Director of Century Wellness Clinic, Reno, Nevada and can be found at: www.drforsythe.com. email: eforsythe@sbcglobal.net,

521 Hammill Lane Reno, NV 89511; 775-827-0707.

Tanya Harter Pierce, MA, MFCC, has a master's degree in clinical psychology, and is a retired Marriage, Family, & Child Counselor. She first started researching alternative cancer treatments in 2001 when a family member of hers was diagnosed with cancer and not given a good prognosis. As a result of her investigations, and after speaking with scores of cancer patients who had cured themselves using alternative methods, Pierce was stunned by the effectiveness of numerous different non-toxic approaches. But at the same time, she was shocked to find that very few people had ever heard of these approaches and that doctors were not recommending them to cancer patients. So she organized what she learned into the easy-to-read yet in-depth book, *Outsmart Your Cancer: Alternative Non-Toxic Treatments That Work*, which describes the history and science behind many of the very best alternative approaches available today and includes real-life case presentations.

Pierce's hope is that her book will help those diagnosed with cancer to reach a truly informed treatment decision for themselves, as well as provide valuable information for doctors interested in learning about alternative medicine for cancer. She has written articles on the subject, has been interviewed by radio stations around the country, and more and more people from around the world are visiting her website at www.outsmartYourCancer.com to learn about their alternative options.

Bernie Siegel, MD, a world-renowned physician and author who prefers to be called Bernie, not Dr. Siegel, was born in Brooklyn, NY. He attended Colgate University and Cornell University Medical College. He holds membership in two scholastic honor societies, Phi Beta Kappa and Alpha Omega Alpha, and graduated with honors. His surgical training took place at Yale New Haven Hospital, West Haven Veteran's Hospital and the Children's Hospital of Pittsburgh. He retired from practice as an assistant clinical professor of surgery at Yale of general and pediatric surgery in 1989 to speak to patients and their caregivers.

In 1978 he originated Exceptional Cancer Patients, a specific form of individual and group therapy utilizing patients' drawings, dreams, images and feelings. In 1986 his first book, *Love, Medicine & Miracles* was published. This event redirected his life. In 1989 *Peace, Love & Healing* and in 1993 *How To Live Between Office Visits* followed. He is currently working on other books with the goal of humanizing medical education and medical care, as well as empowering patients and teaching survival behavior to enhance immune system competency. Bernie's realization that we all need help dealing with the difficulties of life, not just the physical ones, led to Bernie writing his fourth book in 1998, *Prescriptions for Living*. It helps people to become aware of the eternal truths and wisdom of the sages through Bernie's stories and insights rather than await a personal disaster. He wants to help people fix their lives before they are broken, and thus not have to become strong at the broken places. Published in 2003 are *Help Me To Heal* to empower patients and their caregivers and *365 Prescriptions For The Soul*; in 2004 a children's book about how difficulties can become blessings, *Smudge Bunny*; in 2005 *101 Exercises For The Soul*; and out in the fall of 2006 a prescriptions for parenting book *Love, Magic & Mud Pies*. Published in 2008 *Buddy's Candle*, for children of all ages, related to dealing with the loss of a loved one, be it a pet or parent, and published in 2009 *Faith, Hope & Healing* with inspiring survivor stories and my reflections about what they teach us.

For many, Bernie needs no introduction. He has touched many lives all over our planet. In 1978 he began talking about patient empowerment and the choice to live fully and die in peace. As a physician, who has cared for and counseled innumerable people whose mortality has been threatened by an illness, Bernie embraces a philosophy of living and dying that stands at the forefront of the medical ethics and spiritual issues our society grapples with today. He continues to assist in the breaking of new ground in the field of healing and personally struggling to live the message of kindness and love. His website is www.berniesiegelmd.com.

References

Chapter 1

Al-Kayer, Samir and Qasem, M. Bassam (2006) *Cancer Incidence in Four Countries (Cyprus, Egypt, Israel, and Jordan) of the Middle East Cancer Consortium* (MECC) Chapter 6, in Freedman, LS, et al (Editors) Monograph, Washington, DC, US Dept of Health and Human Services, National Institute of Health

Alschuler, L. and Gazella, K (2007) *Definitive Guide to Cancer.* Berkley, California: Celestial Arts

Americans at Risk (2009) http://www.familiesusa.org/assets/pdfs /americans-at-risk.pdf March

American Cancer Society (2007) *Quick Facts on Lung Cancer: What You Need to Know.* Atlanta, GA: ACS

Associated Press (2004) Alternative medicine use growing in the US, *Daily Press,* June 27, p A12

ATSDR (2007) *Toxicological Profile for Arsenic.* Atlanta, GA: US Dept of Health and Human Services

Barnes, P, Powell-Griner, E (2004) Complementary and Alternative Medicine Use Among Adults. US, 2002. *Advanced Data from Vital and Health Statistics.* US Dept of Health and Human Services, Center for Disease Control, National Center for Health Statistics, Number 343, May 27

Barry, Patricia (2011) The Side Effects of Side Effects. *AARP Bulletin,* September, 14–16

Blot, W, Fraumeni, JF (1996) Cancer of the lung and pleura. In Schottenfeld, D, Fraumeni, JF, eds *Cancer Epidemiology and Prevention,* 2nd edition. New York: Oxford University Press, pp 637–65

Clear the Air (2004) *New Air Standards* http://ctapolicy.net/air/

CNN Money *(2009) Underinsured Americans: Cost to you,* Parija B. Kavilanz, CNNMoney (http://money.cnn.com/) March 5

Connealy, Leigh, MD (2011) *Cancer is Curable Now.* DVD.

www.wake-up.tv

DeSouza, Jonas (2011) Chemo for late-stage cancer patients may be unjustified. Chicago: *American Society of Clinical Oncologists* June 7

Doll, R, Peto, R, Wheatley, K, et al (1994) Mortality in relation to smoking: 40 years' observation on male British doctors. *British Medical Journal* 309:901–11

Eidem, W (1997) *The Doctor Who Cures Cancer.* MD: Huge Health Secrets Publishing

Elliott, Carl (2010). *White Coat, Black Hat: Adventures on the Dark Side of Medicine.*

New York: Beacon Press

Enterline, PE, Henderson VL, Marsh GM. 1987. Exposure to arsenic and respiratory cancer: a reanalysis. *Am J Epidemiol* 125:929–38

Falk H, Caldwell GG, Ishak KG, Thomas LB, Popper H. 1981. Arsenic-related hepatic angiosarcoma. *Am J Ind Med* 2:43–50

Families USA (2009) press release summarizing a Lewin Group (wholly owned by United Healthcare insurance company) study: "New Report Finds 86.7 Million Americans Were Uninsured at Some Point in 2007–2008"

Friedman, Michael, MD (2010) *Burzynski.* DVD

Griffin, G Edward (2009) *World Without Cancer: The Story of Vitamin B17.* Westlake Village, CA: American Media

Griffin, G Edward (2009) *The Politics of Cancer Treatment,* Westlake Village, California. American Media

Haley, Daniel (2003) *Politics in Healing: The Suppression and Manipulation of American Medicine.* Washington, DC: Potomac Valley Press

Hammond, EC (1966) *Smoking in relation to the death rates of one million men and women.* Washington, DC, National Cancer Institute Monograph 19:127–204

Helvie, C (1991) *Community Health Nursing: Theory and Practice.* New York: Springer Publishing Co

Helvie, C (1998) *Advanced Practice Nursing in the Community.* Thousand Oaks, California: Sage Publishing Co

Helvie, C (2007) *Healthy Holistic Aging: A Blueprint for Success.* Minneapolis, MN: Syren Book Company

How-Ran Guo, Nai-San Wong, Howard Hu, and Richard R Monson (2004) Cell Type Specificity of Lung Cancer Associated with Arsenic Ingestion. *Cancer Epidemiology, Biomarkers & Prevention,* 13, 638

[IARC] International Agency for Research on Cancer. 2004. *IARC Monograph* on the Evaluation of Carcinogenic Risks to Humans. Some drinking-water disinfectants and contaminants, including arsenic. Vol. 84. Lyon, FR: International Agency for Research on Cancer

Jemal, A, Siegel, R, et al (2009) Cancer statistics, 2009. *CA Cancer J Clinicians*

59:225-49. ACS

Kaiser Commission on Medicaid and the Uninsured (2002) http://www.kff.org/uninsured/loader.cfm?url=/commonspot/s ecurity/getfile.cfm&PageID=14136 *"Underinsured in America: Is Health Coverage Adequate?"* July, 2002

Koren, H, (1991) *Handbook of Environmental Health: Principles and Practices.* Vol 1, 2nd ed. Chelsea, MI: Lewis

Mazzucco, M (2010) *Cancer: The Forbidden Cures* (DVD). The Reality Zone. www.realityzone.com

McLaughlin, JK, Hrubec, Z, Blot, WJ, Fraumeni, JF (1995) Smoking and cancer mortality among US veterans: a 26-year follow-up. *International J. of Cancer* 60:190–3

Murdock, B (1991) *An Introduction to Environmental Science: Living in the Environment.* Freshwater Foundation's Health and Environment Digest

National Cancer Institute (2007) What you need to know about lung cancer. July 26, http://www.cancer.gov/cancer topics/types/lung

[NRC] National Research Council. 2000. *Arsenic in Drinking*

Water. Washington, DC: National Academy Press

Parkin, DM, Bray, F, Ferlay, J, Pisani, P (2005) Global cancer statistics, 2002. *CA Cancer Journal for Clinicians,* 55:74–108

Pierce, Tanya (2009) *Outsmart Your Cancer: Alternative Non-Toxic Treatments That Work.* Nevada: Thoughtworks Publishing

Somers, Suzanne (2009) *Knockout: Interviews with Doctors Who Are Curing Cancer.* New York: Crown Publishing Group, a division of Random House, Inc

Strasheim, Connie (2011) *Defeat Cancer: 15 Doctors of Integrative and Naturopathic Medicine Tell You How.* S. Lake Tahoe, CA: BioMed Publishing Group

UC Newsroom (2010) Cancer death rates remain high decades after exposure to arsenic. http://www.universityofcalifornia.edu/news/article/9291

US Census Bureau (2008) *Income, Poverty, and Health Insurance Coverage in the*

United States: 2007. Washington, DC, US Census Bureau. August

Yu-tang, L and Chen Zhen (1996) A retrospective lung cancer mortality study of people exposed to insoluble arsenic and radon. *Lung Cancer,* 14, Suppl 1, S137–S148, March

Chapter 2

Helvie, C (2007*) Healthy Holistic Aging: A Blueprint for Success.* Minneapolis, MN: Syren Book Company

Chapter 3

DeWet, P, MD (2010) *Heal Thyself: Transform Your Life, Transform Your Health*

Oklahoma: Tate Publishing Co

Evers, Anne Marie (2005) *Affirmations, Your Passport to Happiness and Much More.* Vancouver, Canada: Affirmations International Publishing Co

Living Bible, Paraphrased (1973) What is Faith. Hebrew, 11:1. Wheaton, Ill: Tyndale House Publishers, p 982

Somers, Suzanne (2009) *Knockout: Interviews with Doctors Who Are Curing Cancer.* New York: Crown Publishers

Wynters, S and Goldberg, B (2010) *Survive! A Family Guide to Thriving in a Toxic World.* New York: iUniverse, Inc

Chapter 4

Arnold, RS, Shi, J, Murad, E, Whalen, AM, Sun, CQ, Polavarapu, R, Parthasarathy, S, Petros, JA, Lambeth, JD.(2001) Hydrogen peroxide mediates the cell growth and transformation caused by the mitogenic oxidase Nox1. *Proc Natl Acad Sci USA* May 8;98(10):5550–5

Bocci V, Larini A, Micheli V.(2005) Restoration of normoxia by ozone therapy may control neoplastic growth: a review and a working hypothesis. *J Altern Complement Med* April; 11(2):257–65

Brar, SS, Kennedy, TP, Sturrock, AB, Huecksteadt TP, Quinn, MT, Whorton, AR, Hoidal JR.(2002) An NAD(P)H oxidase regulates growth and transcription in melanoma cells. *Am J Physiol Cell Physiol* June;282(6):C1212–C1224

Calderon, PB, Cadrobbi, J, Marques, C, Hong-Ngoc, N, Jamison, JM, Gilloteaux, J, Summers, JL, Taper, HS. (2002) Potential therapeutic application of the association of vitamins C and K3 in cancer treatment. *Curr Med Chem* - December; 9(24):2271–85

Cameron, E, Pauling, L. (1976) Supplemental ascorbate in the supportive treatment of cancer: Prolongation of survival times in terminal human cancer. *Proc Natl Acad Sci USA* October;73(10):3685–9

Chen Q, Espey MG, Krishna, MC, Mitchell, JB, Corpe, CP, Buettner, GR, Shacter, E, Levine, M. (2005) Pharmacologic ascorbic acid concentrations selectively kill cancer cells: action as a pro-drug to deliver hydrogen peroxide to tissues. *Proc Natl Acad Sci USA* September 20;102(38):13604–9

Chen, Q, Espey, MG, Sun, AY, Lee, JH, Krishna, MC, Shacter, E, Choyke, PL, Pooput, C, Kirk, KL, Buettner, GR, Levine, M. (2007) Ascorbate in pharmacologic concentrations selectively generates ascorbate radical and hydrogen peroxide in extra-cellular fluid in vivo. *Proc Natl Acad Sci USA* May 22;104(21):8749–54

Chen, Q, Espey, MG, Sun, AY, Pooput, C, Kirk, KL, Krishna, MC, Khosh, DB, Drisko, J, Levine, M. (2008) Pharmacologic doses of ascorbate act as a prooxidant and decrease growth of aggressive tumor xenografts in mice. *Proc Natl Acad Sci USA*;105(32):11105–9

Dong, JM, Zhao, SG, Huang, GY, Liu, Q. (2004) NADPH oxidase-mediated generation of reactive oxygen species is critically required for survival of undifferentiated human promyelo-cytic leukemia cell line HL-60. *Free Radic Res* June;38(6):629–37

Gilloteaux, J, Jamison, JM, Arnold, D, Ervin, E, Eckroat, L, Docherty, JJ, Neal, D, Summers, JL. (1998) Cancer cell necrosis by autoschizis: synergism of antitumor activity of vitamin C: vitamin K3 on human bladder carcinoma T24 cells. *Scanning*;20(8):564–75

Giunta, R, Coppola, A, Luongo, C, Sammartino, A, Guastafierro, S, Grassia, A, Giunta, L, Mascolo, L, Tirelli, A, Coppola, L. (2001) Ozonized autohemotransfusion improves hemorheo-logical parameters and oxygen delivery to tissues in patients with peripheral occlusive arterial disease. *Ann Hematol* December;80(12):745–8

Irani, K, Goldschmidt-Clermont, PJ. (1998) Ras, superoxide and signal transduction. *BiochemPharmacol* May 1;55(9):1339–46

Kwei, KA, Finch, JS, Thompson, EJ, Bowden, GT.(2004) Transcriptional repression of catalase in mouse skin tumor progression. *Neoplasia* September;6(5):440–8

McCarty, MF. (1984) Rationale for a novel immunotherapy of cancer with allogeneic lymphocyte infusion. *Med Hypotheses* November;15(3):241–77

McCarty, MF. (2007) Clinical potential of Spirulina as a source of phycocyanobilin. *J Med Food* December;10(4):566–70

McCarty, MF, Barroso-Aranda, J, Contreras, F. (2007) A two-phase strategy for treatment of oxidant-dependent cancers. *Med Hypotheses*;69(3):489–96

McCarty MF, Barroso-Aranda J, Contreras F.(2010) Oxidative stress therapy for solid tumors – a proposal. *Med Hypotheses* January 18.

Moertel, CG, Fleming, TR, Creagan, ET, Rubin, J, O'Connell, MJ, Ames, MM. (1985) High-dose vitamin C versus placebo in the treatment of patients with advanced cancer who have had no prior chemotherapy. A randomized double-blind comparison. *N Engl J Med* January 17;312(3):137–41

National Cancer Institute. (2007) *Cancer survival among adults – US SEER Program, 1988–2001.* Padayatty, SJ, Levine, M. (2000) Reevaluation of ascorbate in cancer treatment: emerging evidence, open minds and serendipity. *J Am Coll Nutr* August;19(4):423–5

Padayatty, SJ, Sun, H, Wang, Y, Riordan, HD, Hewitt, SM, Katz, A, Wesley, RA, Levine, M. (2004) Vitamin C pharmacokinetics: implications for oral and intravenous use. *Ann Intern Med* April 6;140(7):533–7

Padayatty, SJ, Riordan, HD, Hewitt, SM, Katz, A, Hoffer, LJ, Levine, M. (2006) Intravenously administered vitamin C as cancer therapy: three cases. *CMAJ*;174(7):937–42

Policastro, L, Molinari, B, Larcher, F, Blanco, P, Podhajcer, OL, Costa, CS, Rojas, P, Duran, H. (2004) Imbalance of antioxidant enzymes in tumor cells and inhibition of proliferation and malignant features by scavenging hydrogen peroxide. *Mol Carcinog*;39(2):103–13

Rabilloud, T, Asselineau, D, Miquel, C, Calvayrac, R, Darmon, M, Vuillaume, M. (1990) Deficiency in catalase activity correlates with the appearance of tumor phenotype in human keratinocytes. *Int J Cancer* May 15;45(5):952–6

Riordan, HD, Casciari, JJ, Gonzalez, MJ, Riordan, NH, Miranda-Massari, JR, Taylor, P, Jackson, JA. (2005) A pilot clinical study of continuous intravenous ascorbate in terminal cancer patients. *P R Health Sci J* December;24(4):269–76

Su, X, Guo, S, Zhou, C, Wang, D, Ma, W, Zhang, S. (2009) A simple and effective method for cancer immunotherapy by inactivated allogeneic leukocytes infusion. *Int J Cancer* March 1;124(5):1142–51

Suh, YA, Arnold, RS, Lassegue, B, Shi, J, Xu, X, Sorescu, D, Chung, AB, Griendling, KK, Lambeth, JD. (1999) Cell transformation by the superoxide-generating oxidase Mox1. *Nature* September 2;401(6748):79–82

Sun, Y. (1990) Free radicals, antioxidant enzymes, and carcinogenesis. *Free Radic Biol Med*;8(6):583–99

Sun, Y, Colburn, NH, Oberley, LW. (1993) Depression of catalase gene expression after immortalization and transformation of mouse liver cells. *Carcinogenesis* August; 14(8): 1505–10

Symons, HJ, Levy, MY, Wang, J, Zhou, X, Zhou, G, Cohen, SE, Luznik, L, Levitsky, HI, Fuchs, EJ. (2008) The allogeneic effect revisited: exogenous help for endogenous, tumor-specific T cells. *Biol Blood Marrow Transplant* May;14(5):499–509

Vasquero, EC, Edderkaoui, M, Pandol, SJ, Gukovsky, I, Gukovskaya, AS. (2004) Reactive oxygen species produced by NAD (P)H oxidase inhibit apoptosis in pancreatic cancer cells. *J Biol Chem* August 13; 279(33):34; 643–54

Verdin-Vasquez, RC, Zepeda-Perez, C, Ferra-Ferrer, R, Chavez-Negrete, A, Contreras, F, Barroso-Aranda, J. (2006) Use of perftoran emulsion to decrease allogeneic blood transfusion in cardiac surgery: clinical trial. *Artif Cells Blood Substit Immobil Biotechnol*;34(4):433–54

Verrax, J, Cadrobbi, J, Marques, C, Taper, H, Habraken, Y, Piette, J, Calderon, PB.(2004) Ascorbate potentiates the cytotoxicity of menadione leading to an oxidative stress that kills cancer cells by a non-apoptotic caspase-3 independent form of cell death. *Apoptosis* March;9(2):223–33

Verrax, J, Delvaux, M, Beghein, N, Taper, H, Gallez, B, Buc, CP.

(2005) Enhancement of quinone redox cycling by ascorbate induces a caspase-3 independent cell death in human leukaemia cells. An in vitro comparative study. *Free Radic Res* June; 39(6):649–57

Verrax, J, Stockis J, Tison, A, Taper, HS, Calderon, PB. (2006) Oxidative stress by ascorbate/menadione association kills K562 human chronic myelogenous leukaemia cells and inhibits its tumour growth in nude mice. *Biochem Pharmacol* September 14;72(6):671–80

Chapter 9

Albanese, D, Blair, A, Taylor, PR (1989) Physical activity and risk of cancer in the NHANES 1 population. *Am J of Public Health* 1989 Jun;79:744–750

Balch, J, and Balch, P (1997) *Prescriptions for Nutritional Healing.* New York: Avery Publishing Group

Berlin, JA, Colditz, G (1990) A meta-analysis of physical activity in the prevention of coronary artery disease. *American J. of Epidemiology.* 132: 612–628

Berthold-Bond, A (2004) Better basics for non-toxic living. www.betterbasics.com

Ballard-Barbash, R, Friedenreich, C, Slattery, M, Thune, I. Obesity and Body Composition. In: Schottenfeld D, Fraumeni JF, eds *Cancer Epidemiology and Prevention.* 3rd ed. New York: Oxford University Press, 2006

Bernstein, L, Henderson, BE, Hanisch, R, et al (1994) Physical exercise and reduced risk of breast cancer in young women. *J. Natl Cancer Inst* 86 (18), 1403–1408

Cady, LD, Biscoff, DP, O'Connell, ER, Thomas, PC, et al (1979) Strength and fitness and subsequent back injury in firefighters. *J of Occup Med* Apr;21:269–272

CDC (1992) Cigarette smoking among adults – United States. 1990. *MMWR* 41:354–355, 361–362

Cohen, S, Lichtenstein, E, Prochaska, J, et al (1989) Debunking myths about self-quitting: evidence from 10 prospective studies of persons who attempt to quit smoking by themselves. *American Psychologist* 44:1355–1365

Courneya, KS (2003) Exercise in cancer survivors: an overview of research. *Med Sci Sports Exerc* Nov;35(11):1846–1852

Cramer, G (1996) Advanced Research on Atmospheric Ions and Respiratory Problems (*Certified Medinex Website*, Sep 2, 1996 http://mypage.direct.ca/g/gcramer/asthma.html)

Crinnion, WJ (2000) Environmental medicine, part 2 – health effects of and protection from ubiquitous airborne solvent exposure. *Alternative Medicine Review* 5(2):133–144

Curfman, GD (1993) The health benefits of exercise: a critical reappraisal. *New England J. of Medicine* 22, 468–477.1

Diabetes and Health News (1999) Push button, Drive-through, Remote-control society leads to Obesity. http://www.diabetesnet.com/news032899.php

Dossey, B and Keegan, L (2008) *Holistic Nursing: A Handbook for Practice*. New York: American Holistic Nurse Association

Fiore, MC, Novotny, T, Pierce, J, et al (1990) Methods used to quit smoking in the United States. Do cessation programs help? *JAMA* 263:2760–2763

Flay, BR (1987) Mass media and smoking cessation: a critical review. *AJPH* 77:153–60

Garcia-Palmieri, MR, Costas, R, Cruz-Vidal, M, et al (1982) Increased physical activity: a protective factor against heart attacks in Puerto Rico. *American J. of Cardiology*. 50:749–755

Gunby, P (2004) No lighting up in more workplaces, other sites. *JAMA* 271(9):643

Hambrecht, R, Niebauer, J, Marburger, C, et al (1993) Various intensities of leisure time physical activity in patients with coronary artery disease: effects of cardiorespiratory fitness and progression of coronary artherosclerosis leisions. *J of the American College of Cardiology* 22:468–477

Harris, SS, Caspersen, CJ, DeFriese, GH, and Estes, EH (1989)

Physical activity counseling for healthy adults as a primary prevention intervention in the clinical setting. *JAMA* 261:3588–3598

Hay, L (1984) *You Can Heal Your Life*. Carson, California: Hay House

Helmrich, SP, Ragland, DR, Leung, RW, Paffenbarger, RS (1991) Physical activity and reduced occurrence of non-insulin-dependent diabetes mellitus. *New England J Med* 325:147–152

Hoffman, R, (2011) Nicotine dependency and smoking cessation. http://www.drhoffman.com/page.cfm/212

IARC Handbooks of Cancer Prevention. *Weight Control and Physical Activity*. Vol 6. 2002

Katz, S, Branch, LG, Branson, MH, Papsidero, JA, et al (1983) Active life expectancy. *New England J of Medicine* 309:1218–1224

Kelder, Peter (1989) *Ancient Secret of the Fountain of Youth*. Gig Harbor, WA: Harbor Press, Inc

Klein, AC, Sobel, D (1985) *Backache Relief*. New York: New American Library

Kottke, T, Battista, R, DeFriese, G, and Brekke, M (1988) Attributes of successful smoking cessation interventions in medical practice. *JAMA* 259:2883–2889

Lakka, TA, Venalainen, JM, Rauramaa, R, et al (1994) Relation of leisure-time physical activity and cardiorespiratory fitness to the risk of acute myocardial infarction. *New England J of Medicine* 330:1549–1554

LaPlante, M (1988) *Data on disabilities from the National Health Survey 1983–1985*. Washington, DC: US National Institute of Disabilities and Rehabilitation Research

Lee I, Oguma Y. Physical activity. In: Schottenfeld, D, Fraumeni, JF, eds *Cancer Epidemiology and Prevention*. 3rd ed. New York: Oxford University Press, 2006

Leon, AS, Connett, J, Jacobs, DR, et al (1987) Leisure time physical activity levels and risk of coronary heart disease and death.

The Multiple Risk Factor Intervention Trial. *JAMA* 258:2388–2395

Llope, W (2008) Radiation and Radon from Natural Stone. Houston, Texas: Rice University, May 7. Available at: http://wjllope.rice.edu/saxumsubluceo/LLOPE_StoneRadRn.pdf

Manson, JF, Nathan, DM, Krolewski, AS, et al (1992) A prospective study of exercise and incidence of diabetes among US male physicians. *JAMA* 268:63–67

McCann, IL, Holmes, DS (1984) Influence of aerobic exercise on depression. *J of Personality and Social Psychology* 46:42–47

McKinley Health Center (2000) Physical Activity and Exercise Pyramid. http://www.mckinley.uiuc.edu/handouts/physicalexercisepyramid

McTiernan A, editor. *Cancer Prevention and Management through Exercise and Weight Control.* Boca Raton: Taylor & Francis Group, LLC, 2006

O'Brian, R (2004) Negative Ions. http://www.odatus.com/ions.htm

Office of Smoking and Health (1989) *Reducing the Health Consequences of Smoking: 25 Years of Progress. A Report of the Surgeon General.* DHHS Publication (CDC) 89-406. Washington, DC: US Department of Health and Human Services

Opara, E (2001) Antioxidants – The Latest Weapon in the War on Smoking http://intelegen.com/nutrients/antioxidants_weapon_against_smoking_1.htm

Paffenbarger, RS, Hyde, RT, Wing, AL, and Hsieh, CC (1986) Physical activity, all-cause mortality, and longevity of college alumni. *New Engl J of Med* 314:605–613

Palti, Yoram, et al (1966) The effect of atmospheric ions on the respiratory system of infants. *Pediatrics* 38 (12), Sep 38:405–411

Plants as Purifiers (1994) *Aesculapius.* 3 (2):6,7

Powell, KE, Caspersen, CJ, Koplan, JP, Ford, ES (1989) Physical activity and chronic disease. *American J of Clinical Nutrition.* 49:999–1006

PHS (1987) Review and evaluation of smoking cessation methods: The United States and Canada, 1978–1985. Washington, DC: US Dept of Health and Human Services: Public Health Service. National Institute of Health, 1987, DHHS Publication (NIH) 87-2940

PHS (1990) *Healthy People 2000.* DHHS (PHS) Publ # 91-50212. Washington, DC: US Government Printing Office

Rainforth, MV PhD, Schneider, R MD, Nidich, S EdD, Gaylord-King, C PhD, Salerno, J PhD, and Anderson, J MD (2007) Stress reduction programs in patients with elevated blood pressure: a systematic review and meta-analysis *Curr Hypertens Rep* 2007 December; 9(6):520–528

Ross, CE, Hayes, D (1988) Exercise and psychological well-being in the community. *American J. of Epidemiology* 127:762–771

Sandvik, L, Erikssen, J, Thaulow, E, et al (1993) Physical fitness as a predictor of mortality among healthy, middle-aged Norwegian men. *N Engl J Med* 328: 533–537

Salonen, JT, Puska, P, Tuomilehto, J (1982) Physical activity and risk of myocardial infarction, cerebral stroke, and death: a longitudinal study in Eastern Finland. *Am J of Epidemiol* 115:526–537

Salonen, JT, Slater, JS, Tuomilehto, J, et al (1988) Leisure time and occupational physical activity: risk of death from ischemic heart disease. *Am J Epidemiol* 127:87–94

Schneider, RH MD, Walton, KG PhD, Salerno, JW PhD, Nidich, SI EdD (2007) Cardiovascular disease prevention and health promotion with the transcendental meditation program and Maharishi consciousness-based health care. *Ethn Dis* 2006; 16(3 Suppl 4):S4–15–26

Schwartz, JL (1991) Methods for smoking cessation. *Clin Chest Med* Dec;12(4) 737–53

Slattery, ML. Physical activity and colorectal cancer. *Sports Med* 2004; 34(4): 239–252

Soyka, F (1991) *The Ion Effect*. Bantam Premium, US

US Preventive Services Task Force. Guide to clinic prevention services: an assessment of the effectiveness of 169 interventions (1989) report of the US Prevention Services Task Force, Baltimore, MD: Williams and Wilkins. 99–105

US Department of Health and Human Services. Physical Activity and Health: A Report of the Surgeon General. Atlanta, Georgia: US Department of Health and Human Services, Public Health Service, CDC, National Center for Chronic Disease Prevention and Health Promotion, 1996

Chapter 10

Albright, G, Fischer, A (1990) Effects of warming imagery aimed at trigger-point sites on tissue compliance, skin temperature, and pain sensitivity in biofeedback-trained patients with chronic pain: a preliminary study. *Perceptual and Motor Skills* 71:1163–1170

Alternative Medicine: Expanding Medical Horizons (1994) A Report to the National Institutes of Health on Alternative Medical Systems and Practices in the United States. Washington, DC: US Government Printing office

Astin, J, Harkness, E, Ernst, E (2000) The efficacy of "distant healing": a systematic review of randomized trials. *Annals of Internal Medicine* June 6

Borysenko, J, Borysenko, M (1994) *The Power of the Mind to Heal.* Carlsbad, CA: Hay House

Braud, William (1994) Empirical explorations of prayer, distant healing, and remote mental influence. *J of Religious and Psychical Research* 17 (2):62–73

Bridge, L, Benson, P, Pietroni, P, Priest, R (1988) Relaxation and imagery in the treatment of breast cancer. *British Medical Journal* 297 (5):1169–1172

Campbell, Laurie (2004) TV Favorites Battle Back. *National Examiner* 41 (4), Jan 27. 28

Comstock, G, Partridge, K (1972) Church attendance and health. *Journal of Chronic Diseases* 25:665–672

Daake, D, Gueldner, S (1989) Imagery instruction and the control of post-
surgical pain. *Appl Nursing Research* 2, 114–120

Dahl, J, Melin, L, Brorson, L, Schollin, J (1985) Effects of a broad-spectrum behavior modification treatment program on children with refractory epileptic seizures. *Epilepsia* 26 (4):303–309

Dahl, J, Melin, L, Lund, L (1987) Effects of a contingent relaxation treatment program on adults with refractory epileptic seizures. *Epilepsia* 28:125–132

Evers, Anne Marie (2005) *Affirmations, Your Passport to Happiness and Much More.* Vancouver, Canada: Affirmations International Publishing Co

Fazio, V (1996) Guided imagery proven a powerful adjunct to colorectal surgery. *Multispecialty News from the Cleveland Clinic.* 15, XXX. Winter

Friedman, H, VandenBos, G (1992) Disease-prone and self-healing personalities. *Hospital and Community Psychiatry* 43(12):1177–1179

Gruber, B, Hersh, S, Hall, N, et al (1993) Immunological responses of breast cancer patients to behavioral interventions. *Biofeedback and Self-Regulation* 18(1):1–22

Hay, L (1984) *You Can Heal Your Life.* Santa Monica, CA: Hay House

Holden-Lund, C (1988) Effects of relaxation with guided imagery on surgical stress and wound healing. *Research in Nursing and Health* 11:235–244

Ievleva, L, Orlick, T (1991) Mental links to enhanced healing: An exploratory study. *Sport Psychologist* 5(1):25–40

Justice, B (1988) *Who Gets Sick: Thinking and Feeling.* Los Angeles:

JP Tarcher

Kamen-Siegel, L, Rodin, J, Seligman, M, Dwyer, J (1991) Explanatory style and cell-mediated immunity in elderly men and women. *Health Psychology* 10(4):229–235

Kiecolt-Glasser, J, Glaser, R, Williger, D, et al (1985) Psychosocial enhancement of immunocompetence in a geriatric population. *Health Psychology* 4 (1):25–41

Koenig, H, et al (1994) Religious practices and alcoholism in a southern adult population. *Hosp Community Psychiatry* 45(3):225–231

Kohen, D, Wynne, E (1997) Applying hypnosis in a preschool family asthma education program: uses of storytelling, imagery, and relaxation. *Am J of Clin Hypn* 39(3):169–181

Lawlis, G, Selby, D, Hinnant, D, McCoy, C (1985) Reduction of postoperative pain parameters by presurgical relaxation instructions for spinal pain patients. *Spine* 10(7):649-651

Living Bible, Paraphrased (1973) What is Faith. Hebrew, 11:1. Wheaton, Ill: Tyndale House Publishers, p 982

Manyande, A, et al (1995). Preoperative rehearsal of active coping imagery influences subjective and hormonal responses to abdominal surgery. *Psychosomatic Medicine.* 57:177–182

Matthews, DA, Clark, C (1998) *The Faith Factor: Proof of the Healing Power of Prayer.* New York: Viking

Matthews, DA, Lawson, D, Barry, C (1993) *The Faith Factor: An Annotated Bibliography of Clinical Research on Spiritual Subjects.* Rockville, MD: National Institute of Health Care Research

McGarey, W (1989) *Healing Foods for Body, Mind, Soul.* Virginia Beach: ARE Press

McSherry, E (1990) Medical Economics. (D Wedding, ed) *Behavior and Medicine.* St Louis: Mosby. 463–484

Mercola, J. Prayer may speed heart patient's recovery. (From *Archives of Internal Medicine*, Oct 25, 1999:159:2273.) http:www.mercola.com/1999/archive/prayer

Moody, L, Fraser, M, Yarandi, H (1993) Effects of guided imagery in patients with chronic bronchitis and emphysema. *Clinical Nursing Research* 2(4):478–486

O'Leary, A, Shoor, S, Lorig, K, Holman, R (1988) A cognitive-behavioral treatment for rheumatoid arthritis. *Health Psychology* 7(6):527–544

Orme-Johnson, D (1987) Medical care utilization and the transcendental meditation program. *Psychosomatic Medicine* 49:493–507

Puskarich, C, Whitman, S, Dell, J, et al (1992) Controlled examination of progressive relaxation training on seizure reduction. *Epilepsia.* 33(4):675–680

Rainforth, MV, Schneider, R, et al (2007) Stress reduction program in patients with elevated blood pressure: a systemic review and meta-analysis. *Curr Hypertens Rep* December 9(6):520–528

Ranard, A (1989) The world through rose-colored glasses. *Health* 8:58

Rapkin, DA, Straubing, M, Holroyd, J (1991) Guided imagery, hypnosis and recovery from head and neck cancer surgery: an exploratory study. *International Journal of Clinical and Experimental Hypnosis* 39(4):215–226

Richardson, MA, et al (1997) Coping, life attitudes, and immune responses to imagery and group support after breast cancer treatment. *Alternative Therapies* 3(5):62

Rider, M, Achterberg, J, Lawlis, G, et al (1990) Effect of immune system imagery on secretory lgA. *Biofeedback and Self-Regulation* 15(4):317–333

Rousseau, A, Hermann, B, Whitman, S (1985) Effects of progressive relaxation on epilepsy: analysis of a series of cases. *Psychological Reports* 57:1203–12

Schneider, R, et al (2007) In Search of an Optimal Behavioral Treatment for Hypertension. (Johnson, E, Gentry, W, Julius, S eds) *Personality, Elevated Blood Pressure, and Essential Hypertension.* Washington, DC: Hemisphere

Scott, D, et al (1986) Comparative trial of clinical relaxation and an anti-emetic drug regime in reducing chemotherapy-related nausea and vomiting. *Cancer Nursing* 9:178–188

Shekelle, R, Gale, M, Ostfeld, A, Oglesby, P (1983) Hostility, risk of coronary heart disease, and mortality. *Psychosomatic Medicine* 45(2):109–114

Siegel, B (1986) *Love, Medicine and Miracles*. New York: Harper & Row

Simonton, O, Matthews-Simonton, S, Creighton, J (1978) *Getting Well Again*. Los Angeles, CA: JP Tarcher

Simonton, O, Matthews-Simonton, S, Sparks, T (1980) Psychological intervention in the treatment of cancer. *Psychosomatics* 21(3):226–233

Stuckey, S, Jacobs, A, Goldfarb, I (1986) EMG biofeedback training, relaxation training, and placebo for the relief of chronic back pain. *Percept Mot Skills* 63:1023–1036

Study Group of the Association for Research and Enlightenment, Inc (1942) *A Search for God, Book I*. Virginia Beach: ARE Press, p 47

University of Maryland Medical Center (2010) Relaxation Techniques http://www.umm.edu/altmed/articles/relaxation-techniques-000359.htm

Walco, G, Varni, J, Ilowite, N (1992) Cognitive-behavioral pain management in children with juvenile rheumatoid arthritis. *Pediatrics* 89 (6):1075–1079

Whitman, S, Dell, J, Legion, V, et al (1990) Progressive relaxation for seizure reduction. *J of Epilepsy* 3:17–22

www.tm.org (Scientific Research on Transcendental Meditation)

Books by Carl O. Helvie
Self-Assessment of Current Knowledge in Community
Health Nursing
Community Health Nursing: Theory and Process
Community Health Nursing: Theory and Practice
Homelessness in the United States, Europe, and Russia
Advanced Practice Nursing in the Community
Encyclopedia of Complementary Health Practice
(Advisory Contributing Editor)
Healthy Holistic Aging: A Blueprint for Success

Index

AYNI
BOOKS

"Ayni" is a Quechua word meaning "reciprocity" – sharing, giving and receiving - whatever you give out comes back to you. To be in Ayni is to be in balance, harmony and right relationship with oneself and nature, of which we are all an intrinsic part. Complementary and Alternative approaches to health and well-being essentially follow a holistic model, within which one is given support and encouragement to move towards a state of balance, true health and wholeness, ultimately leading to the awareness of one's unique place in the Universal jigsaw of life – Ayni, in fact.